The Fashion Doll

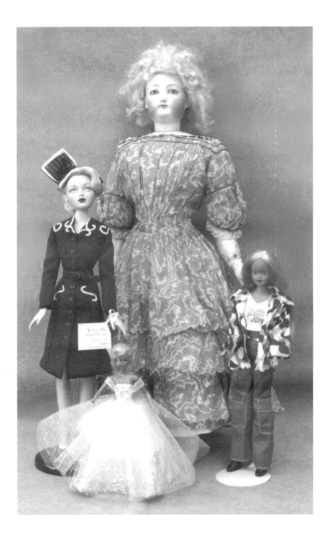

Frontispiece Left to right: Gene, sculpted by Mel Odom, wearing 'Tea Time at the Plaza c.1943' by Lynne Day 1999; 7.5 inch Bild Lilli, sculpted by Reinhard Beuthien and Max Weissbrodt, wearing dress with label 'Joanie Kaye Glendale California' c.1955; Parisienne wearing early-1860s day dress in printed cotton imitating Indonesian ikat; Steffi Love by Simba Toys styled with items from various *Cool* collections early 2000s.

The Fashion Doll

From Bébé Jumeau to Barbie

Juliette Peers

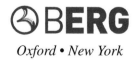

Oxford • New York

First published in 2004 by
Berg
Editorial offices:
1st Floor, Angel Court, 81 St Clements Street, Oxford, OX4 1AW
175 Fifth Avenue, New York, NY 10010, USA

Berg is the imprint of Oxford International Publishers Ltd.

Library of Congress Cataloging-in-Publication Data
Peers, Juliette.
    The fashion doll : from Bébé Jumeau to Barbie / Juliette Peers.– 1st
ed.
        p. cm.
    Includes bibliographical references and index.
    ISBN 1-85973-738-2 (cloth) – ISBN 1-85973-743-9 (pbk.)
    1. Fashion dolls. 2. Fashion dolls–Social aspects. I. Title.

    NK4894.3.F37P44 2004
    688.7′221–dc22

                                                    2004006118

British Library Cataloguing-in-Publication Data
A catalogue record for this book is available from the British Library.

ISBN 1 85973 738 2 (Cloth)
       1 85973 743 9 (Paper)

Typeset by JS Typesetting Ltd, Wellingborough, Northants.
Printed in the United Kingdom by Biddles Ltd, King's Lynn.

www.bergpublishers.com

Contents

Acknowledgements

This book has developed alongside various art historical, curatorial and academic projects over a number of years. Simultaneously material has been informally gathered in the course of recreational activities over many years. In such a complex process of evolution, it is impossible to credit all those who may have, consciously or unconsciously, contributed to the process of assembling and consolidating information from multiple sources. For example the generous and thought-provoking answers sent by Australian curators and historians and RMIT colleagues, including Liliana Pomazan, to a question I posed on the AMOL listserv pointed finally not to this book, but to another project altogether.

Several years ago Professor Christine Alexander of the University of New South Wales informally encouraged me to take my 'doll' research more seriously. Dr Leigh Summers specifically advised me to turn my interest in dolls into a formal project. Professor David Walker was an informative, generous and positive supervisor to my Ph.D. thesis and as fragments of that thesis appear in this narrative perhaps he may be considered to be Barbie's Great Uncle. Associate Professor Johanna M. Smith of UT Arlington has always been most supportive of my work, as has Dr Anita Callaway. Stephanie Britton published an earlier essay on Barbie in 1998 and has followed the subsequent developments with interest.

Specific acknowledgements to colleagues at RMIT include Rose Vera for sharing her art library; Sue Ryan for locating accounts of Barbie and dolls in the current media that I would otherwise have missed and Dr Sophia Errey for her unexpected and generous sharing of comments on Barbie, Blythe and other dolls. Discussions with Kaye Ashton around women and business leadership and Heather Saltmarsh on the history of home dressmaking and household manuals, whilst not germane to dolls per se, informed the broad context of my study. The RMIT interlibrary loans service has proved to be consistently infallible in response to requests for obscure titles.

I am indebted to members of the Australian Fashion Doll Club, the Australian Barbie Club (including founding presidents Megan Bouras and Pam Carter) and the first Australian UFDC convention for sharing dolls through informal and formal displays and also sharing information through lectures and talks on numerous occasions. Mary Kuliveovski and Leanne Vassallo in particular gave access to their libraries of doll books to augment my own. Kaye Tellefson, Christine Grant, Gail Brown, Maryanne Greaney, Joy Frake and the late Joy West should be mentioned amongst many others who have shared my own enthusiasms.

Acknowledgements

Some illustrations for this book were generously supplied by North American specialist doll auctioneers, Skinners and McMasters Harris, when I wrote to them cold. I thank them for proving that the proverbial North American 'comfort of strangers' is no urban myth and that it can even be relied upon. Mark N. Harris, auctioneer, was my contact with McMasters Harris. Through Skinners I also made contact with Dorothy McGonagle, a figure from the inner circle of antique doll collecting in North America, who also responded with grace to a total stranger. Digital processing and preparation of illustrations was undertaken by Liz Richmond, whose expertise made light work of a complex task. The frontispiece and illustrations 3.3 and 7.2 are original photographs by her. Without Alyson Kosina's reading of the manuscript, my errant spelling would have dominated the narrative to an even more unpleasant degree.

Berg Publishers not only accepted a title on the theme of dolls and fashion, but allowed a generous timeframe for the completion of the final manuscript, which was delayed by family and workplace commitments. The politeness, efficiency and speed of their communication via the internet made working across two hemispheres painless. Kathryn Earle, Anne Hobbs and Caroline McCarthy have been my main contacts at Berg. Before her sudden and untimely death, my mother knew that the contract for this book had been signed, and I dedicate this text to her.

The Fashion Doll is an independent academic study of the history of dolls over the last century and a half in public and private collections by the author, Juliette Peers. It has in no way been sponsored or commissioned by any of the companies discussed as an endorsement of their products. This work represents solely the opinions of the author who is in no way affiliated with any of the companies discussed. A number of the dolls discussed are registered trademarks, all of whom may be protected by various laws in their own jurisdictions. Discussion of these names is purely in the course of this academic analysis. These include Mattel: Barbie, Ken, My Scene and associated trademarks; Ideal: Little Miss Revlon, Flatsy, Tammy; Robert Tonner: Kitty Collier, Tyler Wentworth; Horsman: Cindy; Madame Alexander: Cissy, Cissette, CoCo; Vogue Doll Company: Ginny, Jill, Geoff; Effanbee: *Honey*, Brenda Starr; Simba: Steffi Love; Ashton Drake: Gene, Madra; Knickerbocker: Daisy, Willow; Vivid Imaginations: Sindy; Kenner: Blythe; Thomas Boland: Butterfly Ring; Susan Wakeen: Eve; MGA: Bratz.

List of Illustrations

–1–

Introduction

Outside of dildos and Tupperware, pieces of molded plastic have rarely been known to trigger such intense brain activity.

San Francisco Sentinel (qtd. Ebersole and Peabody 2003)

Lou Taylor's informed and authoritative overview of dress history studies, *The Study of Dress History* examined a series of media and formats from which various histories of content and meaning of dress can be deduced. It would at first appear that she had covered every possible forum for drawing knowledge of fashion currently available to the historian or curator. However there was little mention of dolls as an information source in relation to fashion. The omission speaks less of an ordinary scholarly lacuna than of a strange demarcation in object-related dress studies. Doll collecting and the classic artefact-based dress studies share a similar foundation in detailed and careful observation as the basis for the creation of know-ledges and meaning; nevertheless the two areas stand icily apart. This demarcation is especially surprising in view of the tone of scholarly inquiry shared by British writing on historic dolls and fashion throughout the mid-twentieth century: genteel, circumspect, but also confidently drawing conclusions and creating hypotheses from extensive handling of original items. There is a clear parallel between British writers on dolls, Alice Early, Kaye Desmonde, Constance Eileen King, Mary Hillier and Faith Eaton, and the strongly British tradition of classical empirical, artefact-based fashion histories. Yet Kay Stanisland's album of dolls from the Gallery of English Costume – therefore a message from the heartlands of British costume history – is noticeable for unease around the doll's hybridity, from which evolves quaint half-adult half-child fashions and the refusal of the magic of collectors' favourite names. Stanisland avers that there are no Jumeau or Bru dolls in the collection (1970: 3).

Likewise British writers on dolls are at pains to demarcate their field from fashion and dress history. Both Kaye Desmonde (1972: 12) and Constance Eileen King (1977: 331, 336) indicated that the Parisienne dolls of nineteenth-century France were not sources for fashion information as they were 'made solely as luxury toys and not as mannequins' (Desmonde 1972: 12). This disavowal contra-dicts Victorian belief and primary sources. William Henry Cremer, who ran one of Victorian London's most prestigious toy shops, stated in 1873 'numbers of dolls are made whose trousseaux show much taste, and are so elegant, that they are constantly used by dress and bonnetmakers as types of Parisienne toilettes' (qtd Coleman et al. 1975: 157). Researchers currently working with French archives and primary sources increasingly affirm that French dolls were part of the nineteenth-century version of the 'fashion system' in France (Theimer and Theriault 1994: 32, 83). These counter-arguments problematise the naturalness and reasonableness of the British denial of the French employment of dolls in relation to fashion. King further indicates that these Parisienne dolls, the tea parties and fashion *concours* which the dolls and their wealthy owners attended during the Second Empire, and even the doll parades at orphanages and children's homes, are a sign of excess (King 1977: 330). Referenced by implication is a cluster of wider ideas around fashion, the Other, the non-British, female irresponsibility, and the duty and identity of the ideal citizen that suggests that these denials of dolls' use in the French fashion industry may not be as seamless and innocent as their surface presentation implies. Likewise the reader may already discern the shadow of texts and arguments around Barbie, which in these early manifestations indicates that Barbie critiques too are paradigmatic and discourse driven as much as 'true'.

Moreover this disjunction between writing on dolls and writing on fashion is expressed by the publications of Elizabeth Anne Coleman. She has produced magisterial studies both of early Haute Couture as a sole author and of antique dolls as contributing author with her sister and mother. Yet Coleman has apparently made little attempt to publicly assimilate these two areas of expertise. She has maintained the demarcation not only between subjects but also writing styles. Her *The Opulent Era* (E.A. Coleman 1989) is more sophisticated, densely layered and wide ranging in its references than her functional, limpid doll texts. The Colemans' book on doll clothes does suggest that costume historians, 'students of fashions and costumes' would find its content of relevance, but the body of the text does not explicitly address an audience beyond doll collectors (1975: 1).

This book refuses this established interpretative demarcation between dolls and artefact-based dress histories and therefore refuses the subsequent devaluing of dolls to consider the history of the interchange between dolls and fashion. The parameters range from the luxury dolls of nineteenth-century France to the more familiar territory of the twentieth-century Barbie doll. For the first time in a formal study, the latter is placed in her rightful context of the mature lady dolls of the 1950s that preceded her. In academic discourses studies of dolls have generally begun and ended with Barbie. Sherrie A. Inness notes that most scholarship around dolls centres on 'Barbie – the doll scholars love to bash' (1999: 178). She, how-ever, suggests that the 'bashing' is misguided, suggesting, as I do myself, that baby dolls are more reductive of girls' agency than Barbie (1999: 179–80). Academics have wrongly assumed that Barbie was a revolutionary, isolated phenomenon – the 'first' mature-figured, mature-personaed doll (Ockman 1999: 79). In fact it is the 'baby' doll as infant who is anomalous over the total oeuvre of European dolls. The norm from the seventeenth century to the 1880s was the lady doll. By 1955 she was once more dominant in the market. Through Barbie, mature-personaed dolls have continued such dominance. As the following essays demonstrate dolls from other eras can sustain the critical and cultural analysis that has developed around Barbie. Other dolls are here brought 'on line' as worthy of professional cultural analysis. A key objective of this text is to place the vast bibliography of studies of other dolls published by collectors over the past four decades in a more academic context. The meanings that dolls have had in relation to the popular consumption of fashion over the past 150 years are highlighted as a significant untapped resource around fashion.

It will also be noticed that I veer freely between two roles of the doll – the doll as child's plaything and the doll as adult's possession. My discussion is led by context rather than any methodological template, as dolls for children and adults were frequently identical during the nineteenth century and have only explicitly diverged in the mid- to late-twentieth century. Speaking generally, the relationship between dolls and fashion falls into adult usages and interpretation of the doll, although at times both the values of the toymarket and the theories of childhood specialists in education and medicine have impacted upon the fashion doll. A particular tension also arises from the interplay of the world of the adult collector/customer with its broader and more sophisticated cross-references and the world of the child-related function of the doll; the latter is always subject to intense scrutiny from outside experts. The following discussion is not to be confused with that around dolls presented by 'early childhood' specialists. Although the relatively well-adjusted individuals that one meets at Barbie collector meetings and conventions, many of whom have been passionate about the doll since childhood, contrast to the generally pessimistic tone of writing by educationalists and behaviourists around fashion dolls.

These tensions between childhood and adult usages of dolls, and the 'expert' regulation of the appropriate images of body and gender to be circulated to young and old buyers of dolls, extend far beyond this doll and fashion interchange into the intense debates about censorship and pornography that have characterised the arts and public culture in the late-twentieth century (Peers 1998: 30–32). Included in these debates about public exposure to material deemed explicit or exploitative are deep anxieties about child sexuality and the exposure of children to abusive, coercive or inappropriate sexualities. These debates themselves are also intensely haunted by and resonant with other issues about power, autonomy and agency in an amoral late-capitalist world (like Charles Dickens many imagine their adult selves as still-vulnerable children, subject to abuse), as well as the divided and contradictory messages around power and promiscuity spun by contemporary cultural experience. Yet some dolls, such as those designed in mid- and late-nineteenth-century France, or Barbie, seem destined to run headlong into these debates about public decency and the innocence of children.

The trajectory of this book is shaped opportunistically, rather than by any set methodology or theoretical framework. The overall tone of the book is one of an empirical historicism, but a historicism inflected and informed by more recent approaches to historical reading and analysis. This direct, simple approach can be justified because, remarkably, the dollworld, from the industrial production of dolls to the particular choices and behaviours of private collectors, has been an aspect of white Eurocentric cultural experience that has only infrequently been subject to academic analysis, even in the twenty-first century when fresh subjects for postgraduate theses are at a premium. The relatively few fully developed academic publications on the culture of dolls[1] such as Erica Rand's *Barbie's Queer Accessories* (1995) and Miriam Formanek-Brunell's *Made to Play House* (1993) impress by their dense construction of intellectual textual arguments and they succeed in terms of the expected formats of academic practice. Conversely these texts are fallible insofar as the evidential base that both writers draw upon is too narrow. Such judgement can only be made from beyond the academy, as Rand and Formanek-Brunell's peer-group readers know even less of the history of dolls than do the authors themselves. From a doll-collecting perspective these two formal studies have a contingent and narrow evidential base that is not compensated by accepted peer-group validated methodologies of textual construction. M.G. Lord thought that Erica Rand was too rigid in her interpretation of cultural objects around Barbie, building elaborate arguments around the ad hoc, marginal and debatable (Lord 1994: 302–3). The climax of Lord's *Forever Barbie*, itself a unique mediation between accessible populism and postmodernist forms of knowledge and reading, is a daring and seditious refusal of the authority of the academic in favour of overconsumption and Barbie's pink-powered universe; when Lord and two companions leave a learned conference to seek solace in exploring New York's department stores, realising that they do not need to give papers or attend seminars about Barbie because they – Lord and her colleagues – *are* Barbie.

Surviving doll production presents a body of evidence that, rather than holding firm, tends to open out to offer further multiple contradictions. In short to use the richly descriptive but undeniably racist term, knowledge of dolls has a strong tendency towards 'Balkanisation' and splitting into subgroups of exceptions and anomalies. Information about dolls is a volatile body of knowledge, with constantly mobile boundaries and definitions, as it is reliant upon compilation of personal observation and cross-referencing of information sources. The internet has facilitated a more rapid consolidation and transformation of information as collectors increasingly communicate over wider distances, but even three decades ago Kaye Desmonde indicated the difficulty in setting authoritative parameters of knowledge around dolls, admitting that she 'was constantly amazed at the number of new and uncatalogued dolls which come to light, some of which it is impossible to get any information about' (Desmonde 1972: 9). As one mystery is solved another opens up. Collectors and dealers – the latter generally have more time and opportunity to do the leg work – have to piece together material lost when corporate archives are shredded and discarded, or locate material that was never considered important enough to be lodged in public archives and libraries. Empiricism is a viable rather than a flawed option in light of the nature of information around dolls. Engagement with this vast and mutable body of knowledge should take precedence over the imposition of outside templates that do not necessarily capture the subject under discussion. Rather than imperfectly squeezing dolls into familiar methodological paradigms, this text seeks to mediate between content-rich but discourse-poor collector literature, and academic literature that is methodologically assured but limited, predetermined in its understanding of the elusive and complex culture of the doll – more postmodernist than modernist.

Generalisations by academics and theorists can frequently be countered by other evidence, not always accessible through the formal and expected catchments of scholarship. Relatively few research libraries hold a comprehensive run of current doll collectors' titles, especially the – relatively ephemeral – periodicals where information about more recent doll production tends to be recorded. Much exchange of information between collectors and/or dealers is verbal and information is accrued in a similarly informal manner. Collectors' value judgements and classifications, whilst detailed, are frequently arbitrary: why should a doll with 'square-cut teeth' or 'dewy-patinaed bisque' be superior to dolls without such features? Often the scorned dolls are as aesthetically pleasing as those fetching tens of thousands of US dollars. These intangibles are not revealed after a few visits to a museum on a faculty research grant or two, or note taking at a Barbie conference. Public collections frequently lag behind dealers and private collectors in assimilating the most recently ratified knowledges, and often bring in private individuals as consultants. Publications on doll collecting highlight different information than that which would have been prioritised in an academic context.

This text is in effect a boundary rider. The intention is to highlight aspects of the culture of dollmaking and collecting that resonate with current scholarly inquiry in other fields of cultural, social and art history. Concurrently the text is literate in the diverse and largely underscrutinised range of publications for doll collectors published in the last three decades. My own position is also that of a boundary rider, a janus. On the one hand I can indicate doll collecting's limiting preference for narrow, arid codified knowledges, such as current market price or completing a series over more contextualised and layered readings of social history or gender performances. If Barbie collectors and collectors of modern fashion dolls tend to reference more flexible and diverse knowledges, then collectors of antique and vintage dolls face cultural horizons which have, if anything, narrowed over the last five decades. On the other hand I can recognise and celebrate the rich, inward-looking and independent structure of the knowledges and practices that collectors have constructed, and I can validate the cultural empowerment that the knowledges and practices of doll collecting grant to people beyond the elites.

Mary Rogers testifies to the coherent and systematic trajectories revealed by doll collectors beyond the academy (1999: 8–9, 78–82). I can draw the attention of a wider readership to the fascinating primary sources that are often reproduced at length in publications directed at doll collectors. I can also ratify collectors' and dealers' recognition of the significance and merit of dolls from nineteenth-century Parisiennes and bébés to glamorous vinyl dolls of the 1950s: a cultural judgement that gains in perceptive adroitness when placed against the invisibility of these cultural objects in such catchments for interpreting culture as public institutions and universities. Wishing the object to speak, foregrounded, as it does in classical art history, I have avoided the sociological approach of Mary Rogers in *Barbie Culture* as it is not my field of expertise, but I provide subjective observation of the collector scene to enrich the reading of the doll as artefact. This strategy has some degree of ideological validation. There is both formal and informal/verbal evidence that doll collectors resist and avoid outsider scrutiny. At least one formal warning against non-collectors' and especially the commercial media's misuse of a collect-or's trust and dolls has been published (Furno 1996: 41). Verbal communication between collectors indicates their scepticism of both tabloid and academic discussion of the doll, especially body image discourses. Collectors also circulate informal warnings against misrepresentation in the media.[2] Articles about the Bild Lilli doll by collectors who emphasise the charm rather than the sleaze of the doll and her market amongst children and girls (Gerling 1999: 57–61) rather than stag parties, could be read as resistance to the many authors both academic and general who read Lilli only as a sex toy.

The range of approaches varies, due to the shape of the surviving evidence and also due to the changing culture that can be spun around various dolls from era to era. My methodology is always flexible and opportunistic, rather than firmly set, due to writing around the accessible evidence to assemble a text that can display a degree of cultural coherence in the context of other academic literature. The second chapter is a heterogeneous overview of the fashion/doll interchange over the past two centuries. Chapters three and four analyse two particular types of doll product as a genre and as a fashionable accessory: the Parisienne and the bébé. Here the dolls are subjects for writing fashion history because they are closely intertwined with the systems of fashion production and promotion in nineteenth-century Paris and they provide new information about these systems, as well as the meaning of appearances and style in that city. Chapters five and six place dolls in the context of a wider series of historical concerns: fashion, consumption, female identity, female roles and current social and political events. They reference a range of theoretical and interpretative constructions of twentieth-century culture and the key role that fashion plays in these issues. Readers may be surprised that at this point the narrative spins out from dolls to the Second World War, but in some ways any text that references or names 'Barbie' immediately references popular constructions and stereotypes of that era, in a strange and topsy-turvy manner. Whilst some may be surprised as to what urban myth alleges Barbie – a doll put into children's hands by the millions – did in her past life or who s/he 'is', the widespread hostility that the doll provokes may unconsciously relate to these urban myths. Or does the hostility shown towards Barbie create an 'unspeakable' history for a doll in a female image? Chapter seven is more directly empirical and looks at dolls by named designers and dolls' interaction with the parallel, but better-known, narrative of recent fashion history.

Argument is organised around material that is the most accessible. This includes the official information generated by doll companies as publicity and advertisements, and ranges through the interventions made by customers, collectors, parents and children for example in the doll's original identity. Such interventions can range from re-dressing the doll to redirecting or subverting the manufacturers' intended purpose and function for any given doll. Gaps in the argument may in fact be just that and indicate neither scholarly slipshodness nor any particular direction or bias in an argument. These gaps may well prove not to be closeable in subsequent discourse or publications. Information or evidence relative to a particular issue may not be currently available/accessible. Due to the fact that older dolls especially have passed through the hands of many owners who were less than scrupulous in recording documentary information, some issues remain beyond expected standards of scholarly retrieval. Lou Taylor indicates that the exigencies and evasive information loops of the art market, with its 'pragmatic reality of the huge prices some ethnographic artefacts now fetch at auctions' extract the ethnographical object from its context of use and culture (Taylor 2002: 232, 234). Likewise dolls lose provenances and firmly documented origins as much as they frequently exchange clothes and wigs at the lower end of the market where immediate financial gain is prioritised and a sense of the doll's place in art, design or social history is relatively non-existent. The French doll industry's origins and demise, at the start and the end of the nineteenth century respectively, are insecurely documented, although due to the wealth of material emerging from French archives and the meticulous documentary practices of legal process, both commercial and familial, in nineteenth-century France, some further light may be cast in the future.

Fashion, with its myriad publications and a wealth of contemporary journalistic copy, is a far better known and securely documented entity. As stated the relatively straightforward and simple approach of this text reflects the underdeveloped level of textual discussions of dolls. Writers such as Flügel, von Boehn, Cunnington,

Laver, Bell and also Doris Langley Moore provide an earlier generation of professionalism in fashion history. Langley Moore, to some degree, anticipated feminist theory by foregrounding female experiential knowledges and female self-expression/ construction through fashion. Her notorious, yet fascinatingly compelling, pictorial album of friends and celebrities from British stage and social circles parading in historic costumes (Moore 1949) may be museologically immoral, as well as an unpleasant exposé of British class privilege in tying the definition of 'beauty' to social prominence, but it brings essentially private female notions of friendship and the performance of elegance into public view. It also introduces the 'lived' element that is inherent in fashion's aesthetic but so often eludes capture by the historian and curator. The complex level of current theoretical writing around dress and the body or the avant-garde of nineteenth-century Paris is built upon a substructure of previous texts, which does not exist for dolls. Writing around dolls is still at the art historical stage of Mrs Jameson or (rarely) Walter Pater. The level of Berenson, Morelli or the Wilhelmine school of art historical pioneers has hardly been reached. As at c.1900 with writing around art, many publications around dolls are closely imbricated with the needs and values of the high-end marketplace, or in the case of writing around modern dolls texts are drawn from advertorial copy or press releases provided by dollmaking companies.

Dolls raise so many issues about the representation and cultural positioning of the feminine in society that the narrative could be extended to censorship and the erotic, as mentioned above, or ethnicity, postcolonialism and Othering, or marketing, branding and global corporations – subjects that cut across but are not synonymous with the doll and fashion interchange. Space does not permit the exploration of the mimetic perfection of representation and bodily structure that certain dolls aspire to, which cross-references many themes of cultural currency from liposuction to the curatorial reassessment of Bouguereau. The doll's occasional appearance in discourses of the *unheimlich* and the abject in contemporary art is another valid point of discussion which must be sidelined, as too her manifestation in popularist constructions of the 'gothic' and the macabre. Thus for Rainer Maria Rilke she is 'the superficially painted watery corpse borne up and carried along on the floodwaters of our tenderness' (Rilke 1994: 31); for another twentieth-century poet, Denise Duhamel, the doll is no Pre-Raphaelite Ophelia, but the more horrifying corpses of Auschwitz or Baba Yar, 'a pile of dolls like herself, naked and dirty, in the mass grave of a toy chest' (Duhamel 1999: 163). The bébé's ball-jointed body became the doll norm of the early-twentieth century and ultimately a central focus of the work of Hans Bellmer.[3] At the opposite end of the scale to the dolls who materialise as a symbol of the human body are the flat, graphic paper dolls, first appearing in the late-eighteenth century. Their story appears intermittently in the following pages as an indication of popular participation in fashion, but could support further investigation.

The doll has many feminist resonances. Not only does she supposedly provide harsh, reductive lessons for oppressed females, she is also a site for female creativity and entrepreneurship. Augusta Montanari, Adelaide Huret, Leontine Rohmer, Jenny Béreux, Madame Lavallée-Peronne, Ernestine Jumeau, Appolyne Bru, Elisa Prevost, Mesdames Lafitte and Desirat, Lotte Pritzel, Käthe Kruse, Martha Maar, Grace Storey Putnam, Rose O'Neill, Jennie Graves, 'Madame' Beatrice Alexander, Peggy Nisbet and of course Ruth Handler and Jill Barad, mentioned in subsequent pages, have found creative and commercial success in businesses related to dolls.[4] Handler's Mattel is counted amongst the quintessential North American-based multinational corporations that have been – rightly or wrongly – a ubiquitous influence on the international culture of the everyday in the past three decades. Few realise that a woman operated at such high levels of corporate culture as early as the 1940s and 1950s.

The doll not only frequently looks like a woman, sometimes she *is* a woman; in fact she is a clear, unmistakable sign of women's limited intellect, passivity, frivolity. In opera, operetta, ballet and short stories women may even be confused with dolls, so closely does one symbolise the other (Peers 1997: 72–6). Even the doll's 'promiscuity' in her undiscriminating and greedy receipt of affection from those who love her – Rilke called her a 'peasant Danaë' (1994: 32) – and her astute trading on her physical attractions, as her justification for existing, have resonated metaphorically with essentialised notions of womanhood. Ironically essentialism's key stereotype is that woman is neither fixed nor stable but false and empty, constantly shifting, a chimerical illusion, a performance of carefully judged and confected surfaces and maquillage; so woman in post-Enlightenment, modernist legend is primarily a doll (Rogers 1999: 92–4). When the male edits and re-orders the world he is an artist, when the female edits and re-orders – principally herself – she is a doll. These ideas thread through the following as subthemes.

The intersection of dolls with the better-known discourses of fashion is a central point around which the narrative is organised. Discussion of certain types of adult-formed dolls – especially purely decorative dolls such as national costume dolls, or the many dolls that were found in 1920s and 1930s interior design, including cloth boudoir dolls and wax or porcelain 'half dolls' for teacosies, crumb brushes, powderpuffs, pincushions or milk jug covers – will not be actively pursued except where relevant to the fashion theme. One can, however, only draw a baseline or a borderline of an argument with a certain degree of reservation. For example, some could argue that historicising fashion dolls such as the Gene or Brenda Starr dolls representing the 1940s and 1950s or Daisy and Willow representing the 1960s are as potentially meaningless as the national costume dolls so popular since the nineteenth century and particularly loathed or cherished as a sign of the era of postwar mass tourism. In effect these nostalgic dolls are national costume dolls of the past and the most informative documentation of aspects of current fashion may be the mass-produced play Barbie dolls intended for children, known as pinkbox Barbies after their unmistakable packaging. At least one commentator has denounced modern dolls wearing interpretations of historic dress for being uninformed about fashion and retreating to escapist nostalgia (Foundation Tanagra 2001a). Likewise Max von Boehn delivered harsh judgement on those unfortunate, often kitsch, national dolls in the 1920s, 'Such costume dolls have no more significance for a scientific study of folk or for the history of a culture than a modern historical novel has for the study of history – that is to say, none at all' (von Boehn 1966: 201). One notes his highlighting of 'scientific study of folk', indicating that these dolls do inform, in a roundabout manner, assumptions regarding the interchange and ranking of cultures. However, scholarly values do change and therefore national costume dolls can now be analysed as cultural by-products of the tourist industry and signs of economic imperialism (Taylor 2002: 224).

What can one say about the Barbie doll that has not been said before?

Not counting the extensive doll-collector literature by major dollworld identities such as Sarah Sink Eames, Margot Rana, Susan Manos and Glenn Mandeville, in the English language alone there are several serious, full-length academic studies: the richly indulgent, but learned, *Forever Barbie* by M.G. Lord, the more acidic anti-capitalist *Barbie's Queer Accessories* by Erica Rand and *Barbie Culture* by Mary Rogers, which perhaps mediates between these two extremes. Rogers' text seeks to address the negative tone of Rand's theorising with sociological research amongst Barbie collectors and fans, and demonstrates that the range of responses amongst individual women from diverse class and ethnic backgrounds is more positive and empowering. There are myriad articles in scholarly journals. One of the first was by an Australian academic, Jennifer Craik, in 1988; it presented a positive examination of the doll as a sign of changes in women's roles over the last three decades (Craik 1988: 35–7). Various anthologies are devoted to Barbie including a non-fiction volume of essays entitled *The Barbie Chronicles* 1999 and a literary collection *Mondo Barbie* 1993. Public galleries and commercial venues which have staged exhibitions of Barbie or on Barbie-related themes have published exhibition catalogues. Billyboy's *Barbie Her Life and Times and The NewTheatre of Fashion* in 1987 was amongst the first monographs to examine the doll outside of the taxonomic literature of doll collecting. Taxonomic doll collectors' literature around Barbie can be traced back even further to 1977 with the publication – independent of Mattel or toy industry marketing – of the first Barbie collectors' encyclopaedia by Sylvia de Wein and Joan Ashabruner.

There are innumerable art exhibitions and artworks, both positive and resisting, that use Barbie dolls or the image of Barbie dolls in a professional fine arts context. Such exhibitions exist in an anxious relationship to the Mattel corporation's concept of what Barbie should be. The number of artists who use Barbie dolls in their practice across many countries is too large to effectively break down and survey in a context not devoted to fine arts. Among the most prominent is David Levinthal whose practice has included many photographic studies of toys. His photographs of Barbie range from the menacing, such as those showing Barbie and GI Joe in scenes suggestive of sexual violence (Lord 1994: 213, 217), to the lyrical, such as the beautifully lit and styled studies of vintage Barbie published to commemorate the doll's fortieth anniversary (Levinthal 1998). Utah photographer Tom Forsythe is one of a number of international arts professionals who have been involved in litigation with Mattel over the image of Barbie, especially in the last half decade (Nelson 2001: 18; Peers 1998: 30–32; Rogers 1999: 92–4, 100–101).

There is also the fandom's 'Barbie art' that does not seek contemporary artworld kudos, but is content with the admiration generated within the subgroup of doll collectors and doll artists. The artists include customisers and re-dressers, known generally as 'Barbie artists'. People who identify as 'Barbie artists' can range from meticulous dressmakers on a miniature scale, who produce clothes with greater couture and tailoring detail than Mattel factory-produced garments, to resin sculptors, who reference fantasy illustrations to present elaborate neo-Goth, quasi-occult visions of Barbie, clad in fantastical armour, or set elements of Barbie dolls into moulded animal or centaur bodies. Barbie art is a story too, like all handmade doll clothes, about vernacular creativities and skills, as much as professional art circles. Barbie can also be a catalyst to performance art, of a populist nature unsanctioned by artschool or professional training but operating from much the same conceptual framework. Doll collecting itself has an expressive quality and an inward-looking set of value systems that themselves are akin to the scrutiny and care of an art practice.

And if we grant ultimate credit to Ruth Handler for being the devisor of Barbie as a concept – even if her physical form was the idea of Rolf Hauser and Max Weissbrodt – we could regard Barbie as one of the most successful creative products by a woman and one of the most widely disseminated women's artworks in Western European human history, thus ranking Handler alongside the Brontës and Jane Austen in her universal cultural currency and influence. Barbie is a source of pleasure, self-identity and self-esteem for many adult collectors. Many people ascribe the success of the Barbie concept to the informed taste of the fashion designer Charlotte Johnson, who supervised Barbie's first ranges and her general styling and persona. Her love for French couture in the 1950s formed a clear bridge between the doll and high fashion. Ken Handler, Ruth's son and namesake for Mattel's male partner to Barbie, averred that Barbie was Johnson in doll form

(Houston-Montgomery 1999: 33). The Barbie face mould in production for the longest period, the Superstar mould, introduced in 1977 was the work of a female sculptor employed by Mattel, Joyce Clark (Lord 1994: 102). Thus Superstar Barbie could also be regarded as a widely distributed woman's artwork that has met with unqualified public success. That few people other than Barbie collectors know the names of women such as Ruth Handler, Charlotte Johnson and Joyce Clark does not diminish the extent of the visual and cultural influence of the doll they all helped develop.

The difficulty of tracking and overviewing Barbie culture is compounded when it is acknowledged that Barbie culture is international, despite being identified as North American-centric, so that there are many simultaneous products of different content to survey. *Teentalk Barbies* from 1992 – she of 'Maths is Tough' fame – spoke several European languages, as have other 'talking Barbies' since the late 1960s. Children's books featuring Barbie are printed in non-Latinate scripts such as Cyrillic, yet also use the same graphics seen in product designed for the North American market. *Malibu Barbie* was sold as *Saint Tropez Barbie* in France and *Portofino Barbie* in Italy (Mandeville 1996: 141). Exclusive items appeared in various markets for Barbie. Some fashions were available only in European markets, including a series of dresses with various titles that referred to social life and customs in different countries. The same white jacquard satin evening dress from c.1966–1967 was called *Gala Abend* in Germany and Austria, and *Bal au Petits Lits Blancs* in France. A wide range of variations in colour and fabric from the standard North American models were offered in Japanese toy stores during the 1960s. Limited quantities of these Japanese garments found their way to retailers in Germany and Australia, at least, as collectors have located examples of these fashions securely documented as having been originally bought in both countries.[5] As collectors increasingly compare notes over the internet, more about the distribution of these variant garments is becoming known.

The widely repeated idea that Barbie is synonymous with 'whiteness' and 'blondeness' is undermined by the fascinating and diverse examples of Barbies made under licence to Mattel in various countries by local manufacturers and explicitly marketed as Barbie especially during the 1980s; these include examples from Japan, Korea, the Philippines, Spain, Mexico, Brazil, Argentina, Venezuela and India. In Australia I have found dark-haired, dark-eyed, sari-clad Indian Barbies, made with the Superstar mould. These dolls were produced under licence to Mattel by Leo Toys in India, but were not distributed commercially in Australia, so they would have been sent there as gifts. These Indian-made Barbies should be distinguished from the touristic *Dolls of the World* series of the 1980s and 1990s, which also featured Barbies in saris. In Japan and elsewhere in Asia Barbie's face was modified as the smiling Superstar face was considered unattractive (Tosa 1998: 144). The anime Barbie face used in Japan and Korea, and later by Takara for their Jenny doll after their licence from Mattel expired, was thus born. The recent tendency is for Mattel to centralise the design and production of the dolls; they export from a single manufacturing point in Asia, and with fewer of these licences continuing the tide of diversity and regionalism in the Barbie line is currently on the ebb.

Even the quintessential 'white Bimbo' Barbie, developed in Mattel's North American headquarters, may not be exactly what she is assumed to be. Essentialist visions of a fixed, foregrounded 'whiteness' that acts as a lingua franca of 'normality' and speaks to a generic, 'white', cross-class, cross-generational cultural interest are complicated by Barbie dolls developed by the multiracial design staff at Mattel. For example South Carolina-born, African-American fashion designer Kitty Black-Perkins currently heads doll and fashion design concepts at Mattel (Finnegan 2003: 46). Famed among collectors, Black-Perkins has been a senior designer at Mattel for a quarter of a century, and is responsible for myriads of popular models in all possible ethnicities.

The development of cultural comment around Barbie is not solely a North American or an Anglophone initiative. Professional studies of Barbie are published in French and Italian, including volumes by François Theimer, Marie-Françoise Hanquez-Maincent and Mario Tosa. Tosa's book on Barbie has been translated from the Italian and published in English. He has also written on nineteenth-century dolls and his texts stand a little apart from collectors' literature, frequently referencing a wider art historical perspective and judging the doll in light of broader trends in design and social history, more as an artwork than a collectable.[6] Billyboy produced the first edition of the Nouveau Théâtre de la Mode catalogue in Paris in 1985. This Paris-based exhibition emphasised Barbie's veracity in speaking of fashion and social history. Billyboy's claims about Barbie's cultural significance were virtually unparalleled at the time but have set the pace for many later studies. The Nouveau Théâtre de la Mode returned the doll to recent histories of Haute Couture as Billyboy enlisted a number of mainstream collaborators, and invoked the respectable history of couture by naming his event the New Theatre of Fashion, thus referencing the iconic 1945 showing of miniature couture at the Pavilion de Marsan, Paris. Promoted by Mattel, the Nouveau Théâtre de la Mode later toured to other venues including New York. In 1999 the Nürnberg Toy Museum presented a serious exhibition of 1950s fashion dolls with an essay linking Barbie's origins to the social history of West Germany and postwar Europe more generally. This Nürnberg Toy Museum essay (Astor-Kaiser 1999: 60–65) could be counted as another serious cultural analysis around the doll in a language other than English. Berlin saw an outstanding Barbie art exhibition in 1995, *Art Design and Barbie*,[7] in which the doll was placed in various high art contexts including a rendition of the Brandenburg Gate with the columns replaced by Barbies. Barbie collectors' conventions are held regularly in France, Germany,

Holland, Italy and Belgium. The phenomenon is expanding with other collector events and meetings taking place across Europe. Each has a local inflection: Belgian events, for example, explicitly reference the recent emergence of Belgian radical fashion as an international influence. Networks of Barbie clubs for adult collectors flourish in many European countries.

The culture around Barbie is modified not only from region to region but also in response to the needs and outlooks of different age groups. Barbie's function as 'toy' with princess and fairy dresses cuts across some of the cycles of fashion, thus complicating her role as fashion icon. The range of functions that the doll performs means that analysing her role in fashion involves understanding that other aspects of the range have little relevance to fashion. Indeed other dolls have a more clear-cut identity as fashion dolls, although few modern dolls match Barbie's range, liveliness and consistency of interaction with fashion. Barbie has a more flexible and spontaneous relation to fashion than many current dolls who are specifically designed to reference historic fashions such as Gene or Daisy and Willow, or even the recent Jean-Paul Gaultier porcelain doll of 2000 by the French dollmakers Mundia, which was intended as a homage to the French Parisienne dolls of the past using a current idiom. Rather than updating the Parisienne to create a 'modern', porcelain French fashion doll, as was her intended function, and despite her wonderful Gaultier outfit, she looks like a 1930s corset advertisement from a shop counter rendered in porcelain, instead of the expected plaster. These dolls come perilously close to being like Royal Doulton figurines whose clothes can be removed.

Whilst I may transgress in an academic context by suggesting that one should harken more to the Colemans, Glenn Mandeville, John Noble, Constance Eileen King and François Theimer et al. than to Miriam Formanek-Brunell or Erica Rand, I transgress equally for doll collectors by producing an extended text without the permission to speak granted by being a celebrity collector or dealer, a publicly acclaimed owner of the rare and outstanding. Given the strong validation of empirical research in doll collecting, this text which draws upon previous scholarship – albeit acknowledged through intext references – may furthermore seem transgressive as it does not conform to those retardataire concepts of research as 'pioneering' that are implicit in doll literature. I have direct experience of dolls through working in heritage collections in Australia and visiting museums internationally, as well as through viewing many dolls in private hands on an independent basis and through membership of three different Australian doll-collecting clubs over many years. I have a small claim to currency in the visible and competitive world of doll celebrity as my Bébé Jumeau website was one of the first non-commercial antique doll sites on the internet and still rates a mention in links and webguides.

–2–

Consuming Dolls/Consuming Fashion: Contemplating the Doll/Fashion Interchange

> Only the doll remains, like a delicate insect fixed in amber, the perfect specimen of its kind. No sadness mars the joy we have in the doll's 'eternal beauty'.
>
> Carl Fox *The Doll* (1972: 23)

The term fashion doll has been used to describe at least four different types of dolls. First there are the pre-nineteenth-century dolls used to distribute information about Parisian fashion design. Adult female dolls with porcelain heads made in Paris from the 1850s to the 1890s have also been called 'fashion dolls' by collectors, as the North American plastic dolls, in adult female form, of the 1950s, who reflected aspects of French Haute Couture. Mattel's Barbie doll can be linked to this latter phenomena as she was developed through the late-1950s and was launched in 1959. Since the 1990s the term 'fashion doll' has described an adult female-styled doll, usually intended for adult collectors. Mattel's Barbie can still be classified as a 'fashion doll' as understood in current usage, and the term is frequently used by doll collectors to reference both Barbie and her many 'clones', 'knock-offs' and imitations. The term 'fashion doll' is used generally to distinguish the field of collecting Barbie dolls – and other dolls with strong reference to fashion and culture from the late-1950s to the present day – from more securely established collecting genres such as antique dolls, vintage dolls from the 1920s to 1950s, limited edition 'artist' or hand-crafted unique dolls or even the postwar favourite of tourist souvenir dolls. Collectors of modern fashion dolls can frequently be a younger, more diverse audience than the collectors of antique, costly porcelain and wax dolls. Fashion doll collecting is often part of a wider range of interests including fashion per se, popular entertainment, film, cult television and the music industry.

The original fashion dolls, those of the pre-1790 era, are creatures of myth, mystique and conventionalised stories. Even to their original audience fashion dolls had a certain unbelievable aura. Valerie Steele quotes an eighteenth-century observer, Louis-Sebastian Mercier, who was refuting claims by a sceptical foreigner that these fashion emissaries, the *Poupées de la rue Saint Honoré*, did not exist (Steele 1999: 25). Yvonne Deslandres claimed that 'there are no examples of those dolls that travelled Europe between the renaissance and the eighteenth century dressed in the latest fashions' (qtd Billyboy 1987: 134). No one can be certain of their standard format. Were they life-sized or miniature? The cost of some of these dolls suggests that they must have been adult size and therefore the cast-off garments could be passed onto living women or be used as templates for pattern making when their documentary function had finished. Some eighteenth-century, small-scale play dolls have garments of patchworked, cast-off silk brocade fragments. This multi-hued dress construction seems to be doll specific and not matched by other visual documents regarding eighteenth-century fashion or actual adult garments. Some dolls and dresses surviving from the eighteenth century display perfect craft skills and fine details of trim and accessories that would have provided effective indicators of new trends.

The dressing on eighteenth-century dolls is extremely varied. Whilst some are dressed in motley, patched remnants of expensive silks, others are breathtakingly detailed in their replication of the fashion of the day. Complete eighteenth-century dolls are particularly instructive on essential habits of fashionable accessorising. To their dresses are added lace fichus and cuffs, velvet chokers, matched bracelets, decorative fancy aprons, mittens, fabric flowers and decorative choux. Headwear, from straw hats to indoor caps and lace tippets, is replicated with equal precision and variety. Whilst visible as representations in two-dimensional artworks, as material culture objects these personal styling elements and accessories are frequently disassembled when a prized dress is presented alone on a dummy in a museum display. Likewise the best-preserved eighteenth-century male dolls have a documentary completeness with underlinen and neckwear intact. The information on dress practices as a concerted assemblage and individual improvisation provided by an eighteenth-century male doll in original condition is unmatched. In the case of surviving full-scale garments, pieces and fragments frequently pass through private and public collections, dealers and auction houses with little further documentation. Male dress of any era generally survives as a less contextualised and integrated museological oeuvre than female dress. Male dolls in original condition from the eighteenth century are especially valuable, in view of both the relatively weak museum presence of male versus female dress and the cultural patterns and sentimentality that favour preserving feminine rather than masculine relics of dress.

Eighteenth-century wooden dolls tend to be crude, especially when placed alongside the refinement of many other consumer goods produced during that century in media ranging from porcelain to textiles. One group of surviving dolls attributed to the eighteenth century displays fully detailed genitals – in various examples male, female *or* hermaphrodite. Their bawdy image differs from the accepted image of the doll since 1800. The blow-up sex doll, doomed by his or her predetermined farcical and abject hypersexuality to a depressingly monolayered function in life, as an eternal 'bottom', is perhaps the only exception to the expected chasteness of the doll over the past two centuries. These eighteenth-century, bawdy wooden dolls are still fairly crude in their finish and craft skills,[1] whatever their sexual forthrightness. Eighteenth-century wax dolls show more subtle and sophisticated design values than wooden dolls, but they can still be grotesque, shallow, even insect-like with their dark beady eyes, in comparison with the lyrically modelled nineteenth-century wax dolls. Generally, dolls of continental origin – Germany, France, Italy – provide a more direct source for the extreme physical beauty of the French nineteenth-century doll. They frequently display a higher level of finish and craft skill than English dolls, but none matches the dexterity in religious modellings and carvings in wood, gesso or wax of the same era. The language of modelling and representation of eighteenth-century figures of religious origin is generally more sophisticated and 'fine arts' literate than that of toy figures. Some of the most lovely surviving secular dolls of eighteenth-century origin are adapted from discarded religious figures, and re-dressed at the time and since as women of fashion.

It is likely that the fashion doll could have different formats in different contexts. S/he would also most likely overlap with such genres of functional representational figures in the early modern period as the ceremonial and funeral effigy; the artist's lay figure, who could also be either life-sized or miniature; and the religious figure, who in Catholic countries during the baroque and rococo periods frequently wore upper-class fashionable dress, actual clothing made in fabric, which was the handwork of pious ladies or convent studios. Wax modellings of either religious or scientific purpose may also have informed the format and appearance of the fashion doll. Collectors and early theorists have hypothesised that the makers of various three-dimensional figurative images in the seventeenth and eighteenth centuries employed similar techniques and formats even if they made objects with various functions (Fox 1972: 48–9, 181). 'Who can tell at what moment the figure on the shelf becomes a child's plaything, toy, a doll?' (1972: 48). These three-dimensional figures may have swapped functions as they grew older/obsolete and passed from hand to hand.

Texts around pre-1790 fashion dolls emphasise their unreality as heritage objects. The same stories have been repeated ceaselessly without further research. The urtext is from the hands of Max von Boehn. No subsequent commentator has matched the depth of his commentaries around the use of dolls as sources of fashion copy, collected during the 1920s. His lengthy account is virtually without footnotes and perhaps may even refer to sources lost in the Second World War. Meanwhile his suppositions codified into fact as the twentieth century passed. Von Boehn's other early social histories of costume and manners are also widely mined by popular historians. English writers Alice K. Early in 1955 and Antonia Fraser in 1964 virtually replicated his account of fashion dolls word for word in their own histories of dolls, rendering his narrative more quaint, genteel and unreal with each replication. Fraser's doll text does not match the depth and rigour of some of her historical biographies.

Von Boehn's text had a more probing impetus. Writing during the Weimar Republic, his interest in dolls linked into a wider fascination with dolls among the German avant-garde in the early-1900s to the 1930s, which extended through Oskar Kokoschka, to dollmaker Lotte Pritzel to her friend surrealist Hans Bellmer. Von Boehn's interest in dress, appearance, custom and consumerism also links to his better-celebrated, more radical contemporary, Walter Benjamin. Exhibitions and museums in Germany during the 1920s also began to explore and document dolls (von Boehn 1966: 188). The fall of the Weimar Republic seems to have halted this serious examination of dolls and they have substantially passed out of intellectual currency into the subculture of the collector. Mary Rogers' otherwise impressive study of Barbie made the unusual mistake of thinking that von Boehn's text was actually written in 1966, the date of a North American reprint. She too quotes his discussion of the traffic in fashion dolls across early modern Europe (Rogers 1999: 25).

Von Boehn's research demonstrates that the French publicised their fashions systematically with dolls at a semi-official level for four or more centuries. He tracked references to these dolls/mannequins across the courts of Europe starting in the fourteenth century. The doll was an essential part of the emergence of fashion as both a social trend and a creative genre. 'At the time when the press was non-existent, long before the invention of such mechanical means of reproduction as the woodcut and copperplate, to the doll was given the task of popularising French fashions abroad' (von Boehn 1966: 136). By the seventeenth century this export trade of French dolls was well organised, and the display of such dolls was often associated with public events such as the annual fair in Venice (1966: 139). The Abbé Prevost claimed that fashion dolls passed freely across national borders even during times of war. '[T]he mannequin' was 'granted a special pass' by ministers of the Courts of France and England which was 'always respected' by both sides (1966: 140), such was her status. Provincials, including Germans and British, were always suspicious that the French were having a joke at their expense by sending them superannuated dolls (1966: 148–50).

Not only France circulated fashion dolls. Tsarina Elizabeth ordered dolls in 1751 from London to obtain up-to-date fashion information. Catherine the Great sent dolls from Saint Petersburg to Stockholm to show King Gustav III the original and novel items she herself had designed for her grandchildren (1966: 146–7). Von Boehn tracked a colonial trade in which dolls were sent from England to America throughout the eighteenth century (1966: 147–8). English dolls were still providing guidance to American women in 1796, twenty years after the Declaration of Independence, the new engravings and fashion magazines in Europe notwithstanding. Von Boehn published an advertisement of 1732, subsequently cited by authors such as Alice Early (1955: 158) and Antonia Fraser (1964: 43), for a mannequin on display in Boston. Dressmakers apparently exhibited such figures for a fee, with a higher fee for exclusive showings at the client's home. This particular doll had a wardrobe of different clothes including nightwear.

Von Boehn plausibly suggests that the fashion doll as copy and styling guide virtually disappeared around the late-eighteenth century. 'Fashion journals provided a complete substitute' by this date (von Boehn 1966: 150). The English had introduced paper dolls with interchangeable clothes as a subgenre of fashion illustration c.1790 (1966: 153) and they were soon imitated on the Continent. By c.1800 the national tensions provoked by wars with the French Republic and the campaigns of Napoleon meant that fashion dolls could no longer pass freely between countries (1966: 150). Another iconic and influential doll text, the encyclopaedia compiled by the Coleman family, cites the early fashion periodical *Le Cabinet des Modes ou les Modes Nouveau* as declaring in 1785 that it would replace the 'always imperfect mannequins . . . which do not give all the nuances of our new fashions' (Coleman et al. 1986: 259). The subsequent history of the fashion doll whether she has been superannuated, whether she has returned periodically or whether she has assumed new formats and identities is the subject of the following chapters. Has the fashion doll actually 'died'? Carl Fox in 1972 links modern consumption of fashion to the fashion dolls chronicled by von Boehn. For Fox the 'sensation' occasioned by the first fashion doll, identified by von Boehn as having appeared in 1362, still resonates six centuries later. 'Upon this framework was built fashion's enthusiasm for conspicuous consumption' (Fox 1972: 33–4).

If prior to 1790 dressed dolls from Paris were the most important source of fashion information in an international marketplace, in the mid-nineteenth century dolls were direct products of specialist workshops and small enterprises dealing in fine finishings, dress constructions and accessories. These small and exclusive studios in Paris were closely akin to Haute Couture ateliers and their supporting networks of specialist services and handworkers. Dolls even assisted in coalescing the Paris-based networks for fabricating luxury fashions and textile items, as well as pioneering strategies for marketing and promoting French style in an expanding modern marketplace. By the turn of the century there was relatively little contact between the French dollmaking industry and Haute Couture. Whilst the couture industry in France would flourish in changed social conditions and adroitly capitalise on twentieth-century social, technical and media practices, to ensure that it remained centre stage, French dollmaking collapsed into a shadow of its former self. The largest company in the country, the Société Française de Fabrication de Bébés et Jouets (SFBJ), supplied middle-of-the-road product for an undiscriminating, middle-of-the-road domestic market and also supplied subsidiary markets beyond North America. The United States was already the most lucrative doll-market by the early-twentieth century and was dominated by German brands. The French claimed they sold well in other markets, such as the French colonies, South America and Australia (Coleman et al. 1970: 586, 588). One wonders was it a broken SFBJ doll that was given to Eva Peron in her childhood, with instructions that the broken and repaired – and therefore cheaper – doll was not ruined, but required special love and attention (Ortiz 1995: 14). Therefore could an SFBJ doll have been a formative influence upon a major client of 1940s and 1950s couture? Whilst French dollmaking declined, the triumphant international progress of French high fashion shaped the whole experience of twentieth-century fashion.

In the 1950s the North American vinyl and hard plastic fashion doll was a distant, unauthorised response to the allure of Paris fashion. By the 1990s the fashion doll was both a successful cross-marketing strategy between fashion houses, international and North American, and toy companies like Mattel. Dolls are counted among the profusion of ubiquitous licensed products of present-day couture houses. The doll is also a point of access for fashionistas of low income to the allure of Haute Couture. Through dolls such as Gene, Madra, Kitty Collier, Cissy, Coco, Coceaux, Brenda Starr and the *Barbie Fashion Models*[2] – all of which have been presented to collectors in the later-1990s – the fashion doll allows many collectors to engage with the 'golden age' of twentieth-century French couture when authenticated models by Vionnet and Fortuny fetch sums at auction comparable to public gallery quality artworks. Some of the functions that dolls have performed for fashion have remained constant over many decades. Dolls' informal role as interlocutor between fashion and the consumer has been maintained even when their formal deployment as a fashion broadsheet or an early version of the forecasting agency had been long superseded by print media.

The Doll as Fashion Educator

For over a century dolls have provided early training and apprenticeship into the rituals of fashion consumption and viewing. In the 1960s each Barbie doll and each individual boxed fashion included small illustrated catalogues in an up-to-date style of commercial art, totally in line with the style of graphics that could be found in an adult fashion magazine such as *Vogue* or *Harper's Bazaar*. These Mattel catalogues described the fashions available in prose, which appeared to me as a child to be totally out of the world of my familiar experience. As Glenn Mandeville suggests 'even the names of the outfits such as *Evening Splendour*, *Gay Parisienne*, *Cruise Stripes Dress* and *Roman Holiday Separates* describe the envious lifestyle that Barbie represented' (Mandeville 1996: 29). Part of the enchantment was not only the exotic possibilities opened up by the changes of clothes, the appropriate circumstance of their wearing, or the range of garments available to be bought or even the mellifluous adjectives and copywriting, but the child-sized scale of the booklets, and their inclusion with every doll and every carded or boxed accessory. The booklets not only reinforced product recognition, but allowed the child to become an expert and initiate in the world of Barbie's wardrobe. Those exotic dress names became the coded language of a sort of playground bourse. The mere mention of name conjured up the dress itself and its value on an unspoken ranking.

Research reveals that many of the specific details of Mattel's world that currently fascinate scholars and collectors alike – for example the trousseau of multiple outfits, the catalogue with its magical illustrations and text, the presumption that the doll has the lifestyle and obligations of a rich and fashionable young woman, the plethora of 'suitable' accessories – have their origin in earlier strategies developed by the French doll industry. The catalogues published by the French weekly *La Semaine de Suzette* from the First World War onwards for the wardrobe of its promotional doll Bleuette also provided an introduction to the lyrical world of fashion journalism. Each dress was shown and described in the technical terms of its fabrics and its design features. The Bleuette catalogues were illustrated by graphic artists well known in France during the 1920s and 1930s for their fashion illustrations and other printed ephemera (Hilliker 2002: 20). Artists Manon Lessel and Maggie Salcedo are particularly associated with Bleuette's fashions. The graphics reference the revival of the fashion magazine/album in early-twentieth-century France with modernist illustrations under the impetus of Paul Poiret's reconfiguring of the Parisian fashion marketplace and his development of luxurious albums of new-styled illustration (Steele 1999: 221–234).

Founded in 1905, *La Semaine de Suzette* was a conservative Catholic weekly for girls, promoting good citizenship and domestic skills. Inter alia *La Semaine de Suzette* launched one of the earliest and most popular of French cartoon characters with Bécassine, a hapless provincial prone to misadventure. It also developed one of the greatest repositories of historic patterns for *la mode enfantine* with the weekly spread and later stand-alone catalogues of patterns for doll clothes. Bleuette's clothes were designed specifically for her. She was originally a marketing promotion for the magazine, and patterns for clothes in her size were part of the regular weekly content. The patterns proved so popular that they were soon augmented by prêt-à-porter garments sold through the magazine's office and later produced as an exclusive line by manufacturers. For five decades Bleuette with her ever-changing wardrobe was the favourite 'doll of choice' for French-speaking girls, as well as an introduction to both dressmaking skills and the seasonable changes of high fashion. The pleasure of fashion soon overtook the training of 'good' Catholic wives and mothers. 'Through Bleuette, Henri Gautier the publishers and Jacqueline Rivière, the editor, wanted to teach their younger readers how to sew and how to choose the right clothing for every occasion. For this purpose many of the issues include a pattern with extensive explanations that give us, today, the opportunity to understand what was considered as "important" by that generation' (Odin 2002: 34). As with Barbie's fashions, Bleuette's fashions are vivid social history documents. 'Bleuette and her wardrobe are steeped in the history of France. The best examples of this may be the names given to some of Bleuette's clothes during WW1: Foch, Tipperary, *Tsarine* and *Croix Rouge*' (Odin 2002: 34).

Bleuette's albums of seasonal fashions prefigured the Barbie booklets. Although having a more child-like persona than Barbie, Bleuette precedes her by easily amassing a large wardrobe of clothes and accessories. Unlike the ready-made Mattel product, Bleuette's clothing is often a testament to the young girls who owned the dolls, although ready-made dresses were available through the catalogues. Bleuette stands between the couture world of the Parisienne and the prêt-à-porter wardrobe of Barbie. She descended from the French bébé, a fashionable doll in child format. Bleuette partly reflected the mass market and was geared more explicitly to discourses of good citizenship and social probity than the bébé, a creation who, at her most extreme, was faintly erotic and also socially, totally self-indulgent.

Barbie's doll identity as an ultra-fashionable young woman goes back two generations further than Bleuette to the Parisiennes or poupée dolls of mid-nineteenth-century France. The precedent provided by French dollmakers has been even more securely buried in cultural memory than the obscured, postwar West German source of the Barbie doll. Only in 1996 did Barbie collector literature identify nineteenth-century French Parisienne dolls as ancestresses of Barbie (Fennick 1996: 9–10). Mel Odom, who pioneered the first commercially success-ful challenge to Barbie, the Gene doll, also collects vintage and antique fashion dolls. Unlike many promoters of current adult-personaed dolls, he openly acknow-ledges that nineteenth-century French dolls and their sizeable collections of elaborate dresses and accessories influenced his desire to create a doll larger than Barbie, with a detailed and quality trousseau, who owned 'her own wardrobe trunk, lingerie and clothing for every occasion' (Anon 2001: 10). This amnesia underpins an assumption amongst both professionals and the general public that the Mattel product is singular, innovative and without precedent.

Using the periodical paper to educate girls about sewing, and thereby also induct them into the pleasures offered by fashion, extends further back to French popular journalism of the 1860s with *La Poupée Modèle*, founded in 1863 by Madame Lavallée-Peronne. This journal presented patterns for dolls' clothes, as well as promoting the dolls and fashions of high-class Parisian ateliers. The mid-nineteenth-century format of *La Poupée Modèle*, with its hand-tinted lithographs and engravings, directly echoed those of adult fashion journals. *La Poupée Modèle*

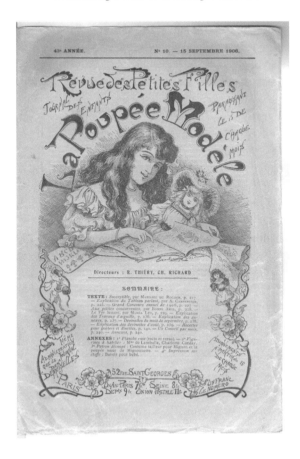

Figure 2.1 Emilie Robida cover design for *La Poupée Modèle* 43:10, 15 September 1906.

was still appearing in the early-1900s and held its own against *La Semaine de Suzette* until 1924. In the early-1900s the journal carried patterns for dolls' clothes in a number of formats, including precut patterns to size in tissue and fabric and also patterns to be traced from the pages of the magazines. Embroidery and fancy-work patterns were also featured and the journal held competitions for doll dressing. The beautiful hand-tinted plates of the Second Empire era had disappeared, but there were paper dolls, recipes, puzzles, games, short stories and a correspondence bureau where Chiffonette dispensed advice on matters from dress to success at school. When *La Poupée Modèle* presented a pattern for a female doll-sized judge's robe and hat in 1906, decades before women were even granted the vote in France, one could suggest that even the speculative 'We Girls Can Do Anything' feminist rhetoric associated with Barbie in the 1980s had already been pre-empted by the French doll industry. However the costume was part of the topsy-turvy world of dressing dolls for carnival, a refined hint of the old ritual of woman on top, rather than a demand for legal equality, but a judge was no less unexpected a female role in 1906 than an astronaut would be in 1966, when Mattel produced a space suit for Barbie. From at least 1863 to 1906, *La Poupée Modèle* appears to have been associated commercially with the mainstream Parisian fashion journal *Le Journal des Demoiselles*. As late as 1906 *Grande Sœur* – Big Sister – was advised by Chiffonette of the correspondence pages of *La Poupée Modèle* to subscribe to *Le Journal des Demoiselles*, so *La Poupée Modèle* was regarded as a preparation for full responsibility as adult fashion consumer.

La Poupée Modèle was shortly followed by two rivals *Gazette de la Poupée* and *La Poupée* also founded in 1863, but of a shorter lifespan. The Colemans suggested that the rival journals did not present such high-quality dress patterns, leading them to be less popular and successful (Coleman et al. 1975: 104). All three early journals produced superb quality plates of dolls' fashions advertising various Paris-based designers and ateliers in the expected visual format of nineteenth-century French fashion illustration. Later, the popularity of *La Semaine* begot a number of other French language children's journals in the early-1900s. Some of these journals also offered a premium doll to compete with Bleuette, including Frisette, the premium of the journal *Ma Poupée*, and Lisette, the eponymous premium of the journal *Lisette* (Hilliker 2002: 18, 20). In response to all these promotional dolls, the venerable *La Poupée Modèle* offered many dolls for sale including two different sized bébés, a boy doll and two miniature dolls. The smallest, Mignonette, came as either 'blanche ou negresse'. Patterns fitting each of the different dolls were included with each issue c.1906.

Not only the French recognised the educative value of introducing young girls to sewing through doll fashions. Nineteenth-century English language journals were also devoted to dolls' dressmaking. A typical extract from such a publication identifies acceptable style options and how to achieve these looks. The doll is described as a real person with choices and needs with regard to clothing and for whose welfare a prudent dolls' dressmaker had to be vigilant.

> For instance, if it be a pleasant day in spring, then a dainty silk or wool hat should be worn. A very pretty one can be made of pearl grey surah or china silk, with ribbons of the same colour or any other that the little mother may desire.
>
> For a hat, a silk wire frame can be made or bought at some millinery store, then the silk is shirred onto it, leaving a frill around the edge. Three rosettes of the ribbon make it prettier, and with ribbon strings – or not, just as suits Miss Dolly – the hat is completed. ('A Few Suggestions About Dolls Hats' *Doll's Dressmaker* June 1892; qtd Blau 1996: 2)

Like much nineteenth-century fashion writing intended for the middle class, a great deal of executive skill and inside knowledge of both construction and fabric types is presupposed. Therefore certain information is not explicitly outlined in the instructions. By inference these instructions are referential to and validate existing fashion knowledges of styling and construction that a reader may have. Such a repertoire of knowledge relates to women's culturisation and experience in nineteenth-century Anglo-European society and has since passed out of currency. So many constructive techniques have passed into limbo that an 1883 pattern from the *Delineator* has to have its instructions rewritten in more contemporary English and simplified by providing extra pattern pieces for modern sewers (Blau 1996: 9).

Magazines promoting paper patterns frequently included information about dolls' clothes as many nineteenth-century paper-pattern companies published doll clothes patterns. From evidence of surviving examples the Butterick company presented patterns for complete dolls, with instructions for embroidering or painting the features, patterns for doll bodies to be fitted with factory-made ceramic heads and patterns for doll clothes. These patterns were available along-side other dressmaking patterns in Butterick's various fashion papers. Fashion at the level of home dressmaking with paper patterns may be at a distant end of the scale from dresses by Worth, Lanvin and Patou for the dolls presented by the French government to the English princesses in 1938 or the naming of a 1950s doll as the 'Coty Girl' under licence from the Paris-based perfumery yet an April 1906 short story from *McCall's Magazine* about young girls dressing their dolls not only advises all readers that their dolls can easily be made to look beautiful with the aid of McCall's patterns but describes the final result as a 'Paris Creation'. Both patterns and the dolls' dressmakers were of North American origin.

The story was explicitly set 'in a pretty village, just out of the big city of New York', itself also a referent of authority in style and direction for an American audience. The ultimate aim for each girl seamstress was to make 'her doll children the most stylish in town' and 'the envy of the street' by wearing clothing identified as a 'Paris Creation' (Blau 1996: 28). Whilst the story is limpidly advertorial in its content, the manner of circulating fashion information is not coercive but built up through consultation and exchange amongst the young girls in the story. The protagonists are presented as capable of evaluating and assessing a look or a garment. These girls draw from their pre-knowledges of fashionable dressing and also consult with their aunt 'an expert in the millinery trade'. Producing a success-ful wardrobe for a doll is a collegiate or discourse-based process. Their 'little friend' Edith White is let in on the process of smart, fashionable doll dressing, but it is explicit that the secrets are to be kept from 'the Thompson girls'.

The imbrication of the doll in this economy of marketing style through paper patterns was clear, as indicated by an article from the *Delineator*, December 1883:

> The becomingness of this dainty turban when placed on Miss Dolly's head so as to show
> her crimps or bangs, is easily imagined; but then all owners of dolls – and every little

girl should have a doll – will want to see for herself how it really looks, and so they will make it up of plush, velvet, flannel, Surah or some other silk or woollen fabrics. Usually such turbans will match the dress. [punctuation sic] (qtd Blau 1996: 9)

This text shifts from offering practical advice, such as the prescription that the turban should match the dress or that 'every little girl should have a doll', to validating the creativity and judgement of the reader as designer and maker. Each girl should judge how the doll might look with such a hat, and the choice of material and therefore the appearance and function of the garment is left to the maker. Again the doll acquires a degree of life and identity. Whilst she is owned by the girl, she is also anthropomorphised to the extent that she has crimps or bangs like any fashionable young woman. The illustrations show an adult coat and hat outfit. The ensemble is clearly intended for an independent young woman in a metropolis, for as well as a full-length coat and turban there is a matching purse. As the coat is entitled the 'Langtry Coat', there is no doubt that it is intended to be a high-class ensemble, with a topical reference to a celebrity and trendsetter, actress Lillie Langtry.

Dolls occasionally appear in mainstream fashion media during the nineteenth and early-twentieth centuries, as well as in specialist doll dressmaking publications. There is a clear crossover into North American middle-class publications that provide information about fashionable style and dressmaking. Paper dolls were particularly associated with women's magazines and home dressmaking in North America. These dolls, such as the Lettie Lane series in the *Ladies Home Journal* from 1908 to 1911 and the Betsy McCall series from the 1950s onwards, who was named after the magazine that hosted her, *McCall's*, became very popular in their own right, and, like Bleuette, promoted sales of their respective magazines. Lettie and her friends and family were drawn by a talented artist, Sheila Hawkins, who provided a detailed microcosm in graphic format of a prosperous early-twentieth-century North American family. This included the delightful postmodernist conceit of drawing a representation of the paper doll's doll, known as Daisy. This representation of a doll's doll was then marketed by the *Ladies Home Journal* as an actual bisque doll, supplied by Kestner of Germany.

The paper doll born in the late-eighteenth century, often known as a *poupée anglaise*, as a replacement for the fashion dolls was in her first decades interchangeable with the equally revolutionary fashion plate and illustration. Publishers and printers such as Ackermann occasionally handled both paper dolls and fashion plates. Sometimes in nineteenth-century France fashion magazines documented new styles in the form of a doll and her wardrobe engraved and hand-tinted like fashion plates. Around the turn of the twentieth century in North America the paper doll still fulfilled her original eighteenth-century function. Chromolithographed dolls were syndicated to many North American newspapers over extended periods in the 1890s to promote a dress-pattern service originating in New York. A 'fashion figure' of a woman in her petticoat and corset was provided with chromolitho-graphed dresses advertising patterns for the respective garments (Musser and McClelland 1985: 30–49). In some examples, as well as the illustration of each garment, the featured outfits were described in the characteristically detailed vocabulary used to specify fabric types and construction techniques seen widely in Victorian fashion journalism.

The Elsie Dinsmore and Little Sister brands of paper dolls distributed in North America around the time of the First World War promoted not paper patterns but budget-priced ready-made clothing for young girls to adolescents. Each dress was drawn as a paper doll outfit and was packaged in an envelope on which retailers stocking the outfits would overprint their name and address; they would then send out the paper dolls to encourage customers to buy the actual dresses. These dolls have been found with the names of local retail stores in the North American East Coast and Midwest. Possibly the originating house was Magnus Myers of Chicago. At the same date the Munsingwear company, a large producer of knitted underwear in Minneapolis, was similarly promoting their products by means of paper dolls modelling the garments (Musser and McClelland 1985: 108–28).

Paper dolls became very popular in North America during the 1930s Depression and the Second World War, and attracted adults as well as children. If drawn by a competent graphic artist, paper dolls were a cheap means of disseminating a colourful image of fashionable style when either financial pressures or rationing of fabrics made it impossible to take part in fashion rituals by any other means. Dolls published through comic books, such as Katy Keene, who first appeared in 1945, were frequently provided with wardrobes based on drawings sent in by legions of admiring fans (Lucas 1994: 11). Paper dolls became an important forum for amateur fashion designers in North America whose ideas became the basis of myriads of published special editions and albums.

Paul Girard, last director of the Bru company, made an unusual link between a doll company and a mainstream fashion magazine, *La Mode Illustrée*. The dolls promoted were not paper dolls, who occasionally made an appearance in French fashion magazines, but actual Bébé Brus. In 1891 and 1892 the Bru catalogue was included with the magazine; Paul Girard advised *La Mode Illustrée*'s readers that his company was one of the oldest in Paris, honoured by three silver medals and eight gold. It had a reputation for good taste and solid construction (qtd Theimer 1991: 123). The elegance and good taste of its extra series of dressed dolls con-firmed the success of the maison (qtd Theimer 1991: 124). From 1894 to 1898 Bru dolls were offered through the magazine as reasonably priced Christmas and New Year's gifts. By this date the dolls were pictured through photographic gravures in the magazine. These gravures record Bru styling at this date, which intermingled up-to-date sleeve, bodice and millinery details in adult style with a more generalised child-like form of dressing and shorter skirts. The advertisements indicated that Bru dolls could be sent to readers outside of France, across Europe to Switzerland, Belgium, Italy 'etc'. *La Mode Illustrée* concurrently offered less elaborately dressed Bru dolls to cater for a lady's many obligations for *petit bourses*, small gifts, with the Christmas and New Year's Day custom of giving toys. François Theimer notes that the Bru dolls were so popular that *La Mode Illustrée* asked its readers to pardon the delays in the supply caused by the overwhelming demand (1991: 138).

Beyond its obvious function as documentary source for later historians and collectors this copy intended for little girls, from Victorian British and American narratives to the Barbie fashion booklets to French literature such as *La Poupée Modèle* has an additional fascination. Not only do these narratives provide instructions and technical guidance, but there is an existential undercurrent as well. Whereas the doll in reality is known and seen to be inanimate, in textual and visual narratives of fashion she readily assumes a lifelikeness that cuts across her actual lifelessness. The boxes and packaging for the Barbie doll in particular utilised high-quality commercial art in currently popular styles that showed the doll as a living woman parading and presenting the fashions as if she were a model. Mattel illustrations of the 1960s show Barbie, her friends and family engaged in many and varied poses and activities, which were impossible for the actual doll to assume or undertake. Memory of my own Barbie booklets from the mid-1960s suggests that a certain frustration arose because the illustrations always presented the doll in a dynamic and flexible manner that reality could not match.

Likewise in earlier Victorian narratives these issues of fantasy and reality are blurred when the doll is given life. There is an assumption that the doll is a living being capable of getting a cold if inadequately covered by clothes, who will be unhealthy and lethargic without proper exercise, who – even if she is a young lady – is also dependent upon the judicious mothering of the girl-owner for the maintenance of her well-being. Early French illustrations, such as in *La Poupée Modèle* or produced by various dollmakers as advertising material, also cannot firmly fix the identity of the doll as either inanimate object or imagined woman/girl. They constantly shift between an image of the doll as a doll, and the doll as a living person. As doll, propped stiffly on a stand, her disjunctive joints showing on her wrists or knees indicate, like the neck bolts and extended forehead of Frankenstein's monster, her essential artificiality. In other illustrations the doll or dolls stand alone and move naturally, just as in Mattel illustrations in the 1950s and 1960s. In one remarkable plate reproduced by the Colemans from *Gazette de la Poupée* (Coleman et al. 1975: 103) the doll walks the streets of Paris in 1862, unchaperoned, wearing a walking dress from Maison de la Petite Créole and she posts a letter. Behind her a poster on a wall advertises a charity appeal. It testifies to the respectability of the space in which the doll walks and also indicates her own class and responsibility. Yet ironically it also indicates how the spaces of the modern city and the women (and dolls) who walk through them were suspect, unless clearly signposted as beyond reproach. The charm is that the scene of unchaperoned pedestrianship through Second Empire Paris is equally impossible if the figure is read as either a doll (who cannot walk in reality) or an upper-class girl (who would not be allowed outside the home unsupervised). Another *Gazette de la Poupée* plate presents two Huret dolls in the upper-class interior that is an expected space for the presentation of nineteenth-century French fashion illustration. However whilst the setting is straightforward, the representation of the dolls is not as they are presented as alive and able to interact with one another. Between them they are winding a skein of thread: the implication is that what we are viewing is not only instructions for styling directions, as in any French fashion plate, but a place where dolls live and function independently, in short this is a piece of speculative, fantasy fiction.

Sometimes there is a double representation, in which dolls are cast as living women and girls and they in turn hold, as their own dolls, identifiable product from the same manufacturer, as in a trade card produced for Bru in the late 1880s (Theimer 1991: 123). Dolls frequently inhabit a world of objects, furniture, plants and architecture that matches their scale, but also matches the visual style of the Second Empire and Third Republic. It is only textual components that firmly identify the figures as dolls rather than women or children, or perhaps that the plate may come from *La Poupée Modèle* rather than *Le Moniteur de la Mode*. In the case of *La Poupée Modèle* even the text does not stand firm in its early years as Madame Lavallée-Peronne wrote text as editor under the guise of a doll. When the doll is shown in mainstream fashion plates, her identity and function is fixed, as is her scale. She is held by a child, or she stands and is admired by women and/or girls.

Drawing Cultural and Fashion Meanings from Texts Around Dolls

Like academic studies of singer Madonna or romance novels, lectures and texts around the Barbie doll symbolise a crude, popular and conservative stereotype of the modern face of the academy and feminist discourse.[3] Barbie generates intense and divergent meanings. Depending on the audience's opinion, Barbie is either a malign symbol of the knowing and ever-flexible strategies of the capitalist system, or she is a source of delight, a symbol of glamour, high fashion and style, a fascinating index of cultural change and nostalgic memory. For both Barbie's fans and detractors she is assumed to stand alone and inexplicable. M.G. Lord's persuasive *Forever Barbie* proclaims Barbie's status as incomparable plastic mystery to defend her from detractors. A similar strategy has permitted the reverence of the

Virgin Mary across many centuries, against the cultural patterns of a widespread disparaging of the feminine. Yet Barbie is merely the most high profile of a series of iconic dolls, beloved among collectors.

The literature produced around fashion – especially from an academic-theoretical perspective – is more complex than the majority of texts written around dolls, with the exception of those around Barbie. Fashion has generally been better served than dolls in professional literature because much discourse around dolls produced by collectors is for consumption by an audience of initiates. Beyond collectors' circles and forums, dolls generally lack validation and are regarded as only having passing interest. Fashion is conversely well documented and enjoys far greater respect as an artform in its own right. Even anti-fashion or ephemeral fashions can boast such cohesive textual appreciation as Ted Polhemus' *Style Surfing* (1996). Yet the doll would surely sustain the recent manner of analysis that has been directed to fashion, gender and images of female beauty.

Collectors' literature on dolls often lacks vividness and diversity of purpose in comparison to fashion literature. Yet the difference in critical accounts should not obscure the strong similarities between doll collecting and fashion. If one reads fashion as a semiological system that the fan or adherent knowingly enters into when s/he puts on a garment and leaves the home, then collecting could be seen as having affinity with fashion, insofar as it is a deeply complex language managed and kept in circulation by initiates. Collecting's semiological system flourishes independent of institutional validation provided by universities or public galleries, but, insofar as its rituals are knowing and complicated, collecting could stand as an indication of the complexity of cultural experience and practice spun by the so-called 'ordinary people'. The rituals and practices around collecting overlap, to some degree, with the impetus of 'outsider art'. Conversely as collecting is frequently a formal, controlled and precise activity, despite its popular and vernacular origins, it was refused the mid-twentieth-century modernist validation of 'raw' creativity that has changed the cultural paradigms around outsider art.

In collectors' publications, many of the more interesting issues raised by the dolls are usually treated as accessory to the fact of more important issues of authenticity and validation or completing a particular series. Often fascinating early advertising copy and journalistic accounts are reproduced without further analysis, or as a functional means to date a particular example. Broader cultural, historical, social and industrial contexts are overlooked. Doll-collecting literature frequently perpetuates much older forms of scholarly inquiry. In particular, layouts of close-up documentary photographs of faces, hands and body types in collectors' books demonstrating the 'correct' body and facial types seem to replicate such texts as Lombroso's *Woman as Criminal*, or early physiognomical or eugenic texts. Mildred Seeley presents taxonomic photographic layouts of hands (1992: 138–9), feet (1992: 140–41), ears (1992: 144–5), eyes (1992: 146–7) and teeth (1992: 153–4) for a forensic identification of unknown dolls. Such layouts for explicating human eugenics, hierarchies of the races or social biology have long been subject to postcolonial analysis in academic discourses but collectors still use them without further deconstruction in much the same manner as did nineteenth-century medical and racial theorists, to establish levels of calibration or authenticity.[4]

Not all doll collectors' literature is so obsessed with authenticity and the naming and correct matching of components, but few books intended for collectors have taken the art and cultural historical approach which characterises the album of photographs with commentaries by Carl Fox, *The Doll*. For him the doll represents a sculpture in human form with a variety of functions, constructions and origins. His text gains strength from the intellectual cross-references and is fresh, viable, unsurpassed after three decades, due to the depth and diversity of his interpretations of the dolls. He surveys historical and ethnographic examples, as well as such trivia as plastic astronauts in patriotic American red, white and blue, available in the 1960s for a few cents a bag (1972: 311), and ephemeral dolls such as a giant Sicilian fertility cake, hand-moulded in edible dough like a neoclassical terracotta figurine (1972: 64). Cross-references cover a broad cultural sweep from Voodoo to psychoanalysis, always emphasising the doll as a strange psychological sign, a shamanistic tripper between the rational and unconscious worlds, as well as the product of the desire to record and document the human form. Indeed, in the late-1960s and early-1970s the doll may have been one of the few intellectually acceptable figurative representations, brought into a more conceptual plane by the artificial and alienating elements of scale and material.

Fox's book gains power from the confidence of contemporary American art of the 1960s and 1970s, reminding the reader of the impetus that America provided to visual arts innovation at that time. The seriousness with which dolls are discussed in his book reflects the then-changing possibilities for fine arts. He even references the contemporary debate about 'whether to include photography amongst the fine arts' and suggests that dolls should also be considered within such parameters (1972: 53). When Fox was writing, painting and sculpture as formal disciplines were being displaced in the hierarchies of art practices by installation and constructions. The doll as expressive object was akin to these contemporary practices. Not only can dolls demonstrate the demotion of traditional fine art formats and media but they easily express pop art's exploration of the supposedly everyday object, and the surrealist recasting of meaning and refocussing of the gaze upon the ordinary and the consumerist object. Fox's text is in many ways a manual of surrealism. He has a surrealist's ability to draw meaning from the hitherto overlooked or despised and to read the unexpectedly conjoined. His preference for analogies taken from such areas as psychoanalysis, myths and ethnography, rather than from classical connoisseurship and art history, is congruent with more recent cultural history and theoretical analysis of art, and demonstrates his text's surrealist credibility.

Carl Fox's *The Doll* stands at a fluid point between modernism and postmodernism. Fox, as art theorist, clearly upholds the central modernist idea that the skilled creator can speak to the viewer through design, technique and formal elements. Despite foregrounding the iconic creator, or even invoking the Enlightenment concept of 'the spirit of man' (1972: 55), the messages that Fox reads from the doll are not the seamless and triumphant ones of formalism, but the lateral ones of appearance, usage, myth, metaphor. For Fox, meaning is situational, multiauthored and accrued when the doll passes through the centuries and down the generations (1972: 55). There is neither 'one doll' nor 'one criterion' (1972: 55) nor even one America: fixed, white and Eurocentric (1972: 49–55). The contradictory, multilayered, picaresque world of 'the doll', where beauty, makeshift exigency and indefinable spiritual forces co-exist, is for him the metaphor of a new, vivid, multicultural America.

His choice alights upon superb examples of dressed dolls in perfect condition. A memorable star is the Bébé Bru from the Brooklyn Museum, New York (1972: 116), as well as dolls defaced and tattooed by pen-wielding children (1972: 150). An interest in folk art leads Fox to appreciate the imperfect or home-made as bearing important signs of social history, the passage of time and the hand of unknown authors, which are missing in the archetypally 'perfect'. His chosen dolls are not necessarily the product of one author, but the cumulative production of a number of hands and minds. The information that he can read from the dolls spans from pure fashion history to a conceptual or deconstructive response to mood suggested by the dolls themselves. Although fashion is of special interest to both surrealists and pop artists, it is not specifically foregrounded in Fox's text, but is included in a portfolio of ideas around style and history, to be deployed when appropriate. Yet only a city and a culture that could have spawned Andy Warhol in the same period, could have produced Carl Fox and his stand-alone treatment of dolls. Both men seem to have grasped how style and history could be encapsulated in objects and their appearances, and how the ensemble production of self-presentation, gesture, accessorising and demeanour for humans, in Warhol's case, and for dolls, in Fox's case, was as significant and informative an indication of the nature of a culture as its self-proclaimed 'serious' cultural documents of a more permanent nature.

The formal culture around fashion is, however, an essential element of the visual appeal of *The Doll*; it is graced by outstanding photography by one of the classic fashion photographers of postwar America: Herman Landshoff. The refinement and complexity of mid-twentieth-century fashion photography enhances the theoretical insights of Fox's text. Whilst Landshoff's models are not animate, his professional expertise during the golden age of fashion magazines informs the greater sense of narrative and dramatic originality in the settings, which moves beyond that seen in many books on dolls, without ever losing the importance of the documentary function of the illustrations. His ability and experience in lighting a face, in highlighting a dress, its line, forms and textures, against a background is recognisable as part of the fashion photographer's repertoire. Even occasionally the dolls are placed into poses already familiar to the observant reader as set gestures of fashion photography, especially within the formal and ritualised boundaries of that discipline in the 1950s: hands raised above the head, leaning against a wall or screen, one foot extended before the other.

In no text other than Fox's is the doll's cultural possibilities, especially his or her place within a surrealistic aesthetic, so authoritatively and clearly laid out. Few subsequent writers have responded to *The Doll*. John Darcy Noble in *Beautiful Dolls* published in 1971 and *Rare and Lovely* from 2000, as well as an anthology of shorter pieces from 1999, is one of the only writers besides Fox who approaches antique dolls with any broader art and cultural perspective. His texts reflect a more classical definition of the function and voicing of art writing than Fox's. Noble's is the authoritative explicating voice of Bernard Berenson or Kenneth Clark, adept in the surface elegance of the best empirical connoisseurship, more firm and formalised than Carl Fox in his address to the audience.

Noble explicates the dolls under discussion in relation to established points of reference of art, social and fashion history, but frequently assumes that his audience, while briefed in doll lore, is less familiar with wider paradigms in art and social history. One can partly excuse the *ex cathedra* voicing that Noble employs. He has been at the vanguard of modern institutional and curatorial validation of dolls. Closely associated with Marguerite Fawdry in founding Pollock's Toy Museum in London in the 1950s, he was later the first professional curator appointed to a doll and toy collection in a North American public gallery (Noble 2000: 126). In the context of the narrow focus of collector literature and interpretation of material culture, his position, historically, would have been one of a greater cultural literacy than many fellow doll collectors. Thus he particularly pleads for the primacy of the informational value of dolls that survive as complete units from the past, rather than dolls that have been restored or altered by later collectors. Whilst he cherishes the rare and beautiful with the minute judgmental finesse of an 'opera queen', he surprisingly validates the less than perfect item with original ensemble and accessories intact. Noble disobeys the one-dimensional compulsion for the collector to demand only the perfect and complete when he suggests that the 'perfection', for which a sensitive, knowing collector should aim, is neither crispness nor cleanliness but the authority of an unbroken, unmediated descent from the past, the veracity as witness (Noble 1971: 81, 137, 204–5).

More recently, Stuart Holbrook, in his volume *The Doll as Art*, also takes the relatively rare step of asking collectors to pause and consider the aesthetic potential of their dolls. His texts operate from within collector-speak and its hierarchical values. Holbrook's plea in the 1990s for the doll to be considered as art by a wider audience suggests that, despite changing tastes in both high art and popular culture, no one has taken up the avant-garde, surrealist challenge posed nearly three decades ago by Fox. Holbrook, like Noble, upholds classical connoisseurship. There are no hints of the strange, disquieting or battered dolls celebrated by Fox. The dolls are presented with superlative photography, intended to explicate or expose the beauty of the dolls. Its audience may be 'embarking on their first exposure to antique dolls . . . an awakening to the beauty of the art form' (Holbrook 1990: 3): surely an investment prospectus.[5]

The sumptuous formality of Holbrook's albums suggests a particularly North American manner of viewing nineteenth-century decorative arts and design as part of a lush, but ordered, classical *mise en scène*, drawn from such magazines as *The World of Interiors* and the increasingly transatlantic *Connoisseur*. The dolls speak of high aesthetics but also of monetary value and security. It is a style that is somewhat unsuccessfully mimicked by the Franklin Mint with their constructed collectables for a more bourgeois marketplace. Holbrook's texts are intended to speak to those who, while unfamiliar with dolls, know the difference between the authentic and the pastiche, and can afford to execute their judgement when making purchases. In *The Doll as Art* and *The World of Interiors*, nineteenth-century style becomes a sign in itself of reliability and status. Any hint of lushness, surrealistic strangeness or even bordelloesque excess that the dolls and their settings may suggest is carefully ignored. Individual items are subsumed to speak through a concerted impression of wealth.

The works of American fashion designers such as Oscar de la Renta or Oleg Cassini also speak to this same domestic market of high-quality formality. Nolan Miller, in replicating this milieu for television soap opera, turns it slightly towards camp and self-parodic farce. If Miller's designs are a lower-class pastiche, he follows his betters with a wide range of semiotic references to 'the past' in costume from the Victorian to the 1950s: lace overlays, swirling trains, sleeve and neckline details, beading and embroideries; this sumptuousness exists more as an indication of 'the past' in general terms and its Otherness and 'specialness', to indict our own 'lacks' rather than for any technically precise or informative reasons. If one can link *The Doll as Art* to the lavishness of the Victorian upper-class past-as-sign in North American and international culture, this lush, gestural homage to the past as surface replication frequently crosses over into Barbie, who has been dressed by both Miller and de la Renta.

Like tourists, academics tripping into dollworld on a research grant or a brief residency in a public museum frequently only hear half the story. *Made to Play House* by Formanek-Brunell, for example, is undercut by the fact that the author's key assertions can be problematised and shifted by other primary sources. She seeks to theorise a gender divide within dollmaking, suggesting that certain formats, materials and characterisations indicate a gendered outlook in dollmakers and designers. Women's dolls are 'soft', indicating a 'preference for individual craftsmanship' and a consideration of the players rather than the product. Men's doll production inclines towards mechanisation, 'realism' and 'scientific management'. In dollmaking the male viewpoint also dismembered the woman and focussed on parts rather than the whole (Formanek-Brunell 1993: 2–3). Formanek-Brunell's arguments are upheld in a more recent, intellectually aware, high-profile examination of the history of mechanical dolls (Wood 2002: 142).

Yet if women made complete dolls as a holistic act of creation, paralleling female biology and maternity, then what could one say about Emile-Louis Jumeau, who was proud of not only his ability to control the whole industrial process of the production of the doll but also asserted the completeness and perfection of his paternity/maternity. If men made dolls that were hard and unresponsive in their materials and technological in their hardness of surface, what of Leon Casimir Bru's soft, leather-bodied bébés (albeit coupled to bisque heads)? Bru believed that his soft-bodied dolls were superior to the hard bodies of the Jumeau dolls (Theimer 1991: 67). What too of the legions of bisque reproduction dolls made almost exclusively by women? Many of these 'reproduction' dolls from the 1970s and 1980s, made and designed by women, featured a ceramic body even harder, more unresponsive and resistant to embrace and mothering than the original bodies, cloth, leather and jointed papier mâché of the nineteenth-century dolls. As these dolls were entirely produced from ceramic, they were not intended for rough play. Some current home-based dollmakers make – and deal in – ceramic parts of dolls or even 'greenware', fragmentary parts of bodies cast in porcelain slip to be fired hard, decorated by the collector and then made up into a complete doll. Again the majority of these makers dealing in ceramic doll body parts are women.

Primary sources around dollmaking do not entirely support the thesis that men make outward dolls, concerned with appearances, glamour and novelty, with mechanical invention overwriting female birthing and women make inward dolls, that represent and reinscribe maternity and domesticity. Seeking to place dolls with a firmly constructed gender theory academics such as Formanek-Brunell suggest that nineteenth century doll making replicated the first wave feminist vision of mothering and family values driving the public sphere (1993: 3–4). However, the most dramatic technical advances in doll construction and the most extravagant placement of the doll as an object of beauty, serving the gaze and visual pleasure rather than domestic duty, can be credited to women not men. If men could be characterised as obsessed with making a doll that was non-nurturing, that was outward, focussed upon physical elaboration and technical innovation, then what of the fact that the development of the luxury doll fashion industry in the nineteenth century was entirely due to the creative efforts of two specific middle-class women: Augusta Montanari (Hillier 1985: 83–91), a middle-class English woman married to a Corsican resident in London, and an earnest French spinster, that most unlikely of all women of culture, Adelaide Huret?

Montanari expanded the physical and theoretical possibilities of nineteenth-century dollmaking when her expensive dressed wax dolls received a gold medal at the 1851 Great Exhibition. This medal was an unprecedented honour, presenting dolls as equal in concept and appearance to the other industrial and artistic show-pieces on display. Concurrently, in Paris Adelaide Huret patented her improved doll in December 1850 and within the next year, similarly to Montanari, overturned the accepted standards of the doll industry with a porcelain doll dressed in Parisian couture. These luxury dolls' consciously beautiful appearances were intended to improve upon the stylised, relatively crude and folkloric doll formats of pre-1850. The elaboration of the dress and accessories in the luxury doll was always the target for anxieties about a non-maternal identity and function for women. This tension between differing functions of the doll as maternal trainer for domestic duties and the superficiality of the luxury doll, whose raison d'être is to wear glorious clothes, is long-standing. It shadows the era of dollmaking and marketing under discussion here. This tension is explicitly about fashion, as an entity named 'fashion' is frequently invoked as the opposite to, and a perversion of, women's essential nature. 'Fashion' is frequently identified as the force that alienates girls/women from mothering. In recent years Barbie has been reviled as the fifth columnist of training women/girls to this false identity of fashion.

The Doll as Fashion Interlocutor

One of the most important issues that runs through this book is how dolls can provide evidence about non-direct, or outsider, participation in fashion culture and rituals. Especially from the 1950s onwards, dolls have been a key means of engagement with elite styling for spectators who cannot access the world of high fashion so frequently celebrated in various forms of media. With the development of electronic media this lack of access has become perhaps even more melancholy because Haute Couture has become more visible, even while its 'death' has been regularly predicted since the 1960s. The melancholy of the impossibility of accessing the 'real' items, except perhaps through blockbuster exhibitions at public galleries, has increased proportionally as the spectacle of Haute Couture has become more fantastic and extreme. Haute Couture's association with the tabloid worlds of celebrity-watching and the star system has brought top-level designer fashion into the texture of everyday life. Parallel to the ever-growing visibility of the impossible-to-afford Haute Couture in such mundane contexts as the final minutes of the evening television news or in commuter newspapers on evening trains, dolls provide accessibility and entrée into this ubiquitous promised world of ideal glamour.

Sometimes the access to fashion provided by a doll is very direct. Couture houses have designed dolls either for charity such as the Barbies provided by Westwood in 1998 and Lacroix in 1999 for the Austrian annual Lifeball Aids fundraising event, or for a one-off event such as the collection of couture Barbies commissioned from major French and Italian houses by Billyboy for his Nouveau Théâtre de La Mode in 1985. Sometimes the dolls celebrate specific anniversaries, such as the later series of couture Barbies, including Armani and Lacroix as well as younger European designers, for the Galeries Lafayette department store in 1999 as a tribute to Barbie's fortieth anniversary. Other doll makers similarly make product available to major international designers for fundraising projects, such as the Robert Tonner fashion dolls that were dressed for the London-based *Dolls Against Addiction* exhibitions in 1998 and 1999 by designers including Donatella Versace, Ralph Lauren, John Galliano and Oscar de la Renta. Couture houses have increasingly collaborated on dolls as commercial licensed items, such as the two Dior Barbies or the Givenchy Barbie. The house of Dior licensed a modern Barbie in a Gianfranco Ferre evening dress in 1995, and in 1996, a reproduction of the ensemble Bar from the debut show of 1947 as a fiftieth anniversary tribute to Dior and the New Look. Givenchy Barbie wears a similar reproduction of a vintage garment, a 1956 evening dress in Barbie size.

Many dolls are now created in series directly replicating fashion history. Notable examples include Madame Alexander's survey of American Designers, *Madame Alexander Celebrates American Design*, a collaboration with the Council of Fashion Designers of America (CFDA), 2000, the Barbie *Great Eras* and *Great Fashions of the Twentieth Century*, which replicated fashion from Ancient Egypt to the present (both Mattel series were issued sequentially throughout the 1990s), Robert Tonner's series in which his doll Tyler revisits the 1946 Théâtre de la Mode, or the French Pixi series of small plastic figures produced in the 1980s of scale models of French Haute Couture from Worth onwards. Barbie's *Great Fashions of the Twentieth Century*, with a doll for every decade, is particularly witty and well informed, more deeply thought through and thematically focussed than the earlier airheaded, eclectic *Great Eras* series. The latter also featured historic fashions, suggesting that Mattel believes that its adult audience is well informed about fashion history. These various dolls directly make archetypal 'Haute Couture' available to an audience that would never hope to be invited to a parade, nor could afford to buy fitted Haute Couture. Many buyers of these dolls with couture labels explicitly indicate that they will never buy a 'real' dress from the designer, but they can own the outfit through Barbie. With the licensed dolls, it is not only the garment but the archetypal image of the particular house that is acquired with the doll. The familiar Mattel pinkbox is substituted for an approved presentation. The silver box of the first Dior doll resembles packaging for Dior shoes and perfume, and uses familiar graphics already recognisable to those in the know. The associated publicity material, including a booklet packaged with the doll, promotes the house and its history. Likewise Givenchy Barbie's box is not hot pink but sober navy and again includes the recognisable logos. Many collectors treasure Barbie because she unlocks or represents the world of high fashion otherwise beyond their budget and lifestyle.

In late 2001 North American designers and manufacturers explicitly recognised that buying fashion dolls is a substitute for buying Haute Couture. However instead of suggesting that it is collectors' poverty rather than their will that compels them to buy a doll rather than going to Paris for fittings in a celebrity atelier, it is implied that lifestyles of the present era preclude the wearing of elegant couture.

> In today's era of casual styles, fashion dolls can help fulfil our need for elegance. 'I think that collectors can enjoy vicariously living through their dolls' says Robert [Tonner]. 'whilst people may like the art of high fashion, the art does not translate to their everyday lives'. (Sherman 2001: 39)

Thus the doll can perform a proxy function like the dolls that Chinese women supposedly took to doctors to indicate where they were feeling pain, rather than undress in front of a doctor. Or is the doll a sort of reverse portrait of Dorian Gray? She eternally keeps up high standards of elegance and accessorising whilst her owner degenerates into a slough of ever more heinous and sloppy crimes against fashion, which are explicitly marked on and shown through the owner's self-presentation, if not her body and soul. In the reiterated statements by North American doll designers in late-2001 about the impossibility of reconciling Haute Couture and modern lifestyle, the grounds for the passing of Haute Couture from the world of the modern woman are subtly varied. In some cases it is simple nostalgia with concomitant inferred critique of the decadence and slipping standards of the present.

> Susan [Wakeen] says that the elegance and sophistication of fashion dolls seems to fulfil a need for something that our complex yet casual era lacks. She suspects our interest in their wonderful ensembles might represent our inner yearnings for a display of femininity and glamour, the time to luxuriate in special occasions. She's happy to help fulfil our needs. (Sanderson 2001: 41)

A more sophisticated interpretation of the impossibility of Haute Couture in the twenty-first century is given by Mel Odom, who displays a more complex awareness of social history, women's history, fashion, camp and sexuality. In his opinion not just casualisation precludes women from keeping up with Haute Couture, but changing values in female desires and expectations. After feminism, women would be unhappy to go back to the old role models and dress formats.

> Mel says that today's women are lucky that they can enjoy such fashions from afar. 'When people say they would like to dress like Gene and Madra, I usually think "you wouldn't if you had to endure the discomfortable support garments that women had to wear with such clothes",' says Mel. 'Women are less willing to suffer for beauty these days. The exception to this seems to be shoes. Women will suffer for beautiful shoes.' (Mathews 2001: 47)

Whilst acknowledging that feminist protest and gains have created strong women who are no longer dupes or care to play the masochistic games of couture past, save the arch-fetishistic exception of the shoe (and possibly Manolo Blahnik's creations in particular), Mel Odom also speaks *ex cathedra* exactly in the manner of Dior dictating the season's line.

Conversely, for doll designer Sandra Bilotto feminism, rather than empowering women against supposedly debilitating and grotesque fashion, has denied them the opportunity to be 'beautiful' and 'feminine'. This missing opportunity to explore feminine values is then supplied by dolls. Morally dolls stand as correction of social mistakes rather than the informed licence offered by Odom's dolls.

> 'Women are tired of being de-feminised and looking like the opposite sex,' she says 'they want to reclaim their femininity.'
>
> These dolls clearly have. They are nothing if not feminine . . . [they] wear clothing that reflects their personalities in a very feminine way.' (Marks 2001: 50)

The Butterfly Ring set of dolls comes with a storyline about women transforming their lives through passing 'self-esteem trials'. This storyline stands as an explicit answer to the criticism that fashion dolls impose an alien stereotype upon women or debilitate their sense of purpose and self-reliance. 'Today they have all become confident, successful women. The symbolism is unmistakable. These seven emerged from their cocoons, transforming them into beautiful butterflies, and that's the intrigue of this collection' (Marks 2001: 50). Thus fashion has a new currency as a visible symbol of the self-help industry, but has not the story of 'the dress' as agent of female empowerment, by revealing the 'real' character underneath the erroneous, dowdy disguise, been a fantasy as long ago as Perrault's *Cinderella*, 1697, and as recently as *Sabrina*, 1954, 1995, *Funny Face*, 1957 or *Pretty Woman*, 1990?

The dense self-reflexiveness of these combined statements made by designers of fashion dolls to validate their approach to their product, and the relative currency of these statements upon dolls and fashion even as my own narrative is being compiled, suggests that some collectors' fears that the genre of fashion dolls is in 'danger' may be right. Perhaps the hyperactivity and rapid development of new products and new (and ever more exaggerated) characterisations in the fashion doll arena will implode under all this frenetic activity. However such an implosion becomes less likely when one considers that the 'fashion doll' is far older than the recent phenomenon of vinyl adult-shaped dolls from the 1990s onwards. The advertorial and promotional texts from doll designers quoted above demonstrate the richness of the metaphorical discussion about women, image and dress provided by dolls. One can see particularly how dolls offer comments around the incarnations of fashion in the current era.

Dolls are viable sources of vernacular commentaries about the role of fashion in women's lives and the multiplicities of possible meanings that fashion can have not only amongst the initiates at the centre, but also for the marginal and liminal consumer. Some of the particular energies of these comments – the longing for a feminine, elegant and passive past, the regrets/anxieties about a workaday and casualised present – may have a particular relevance to cultural expressions and experiences in North America. Indeed an intercultural perspective could best unpick these issues and would take the subject of discussion out far wider. However in terms of cultural influence and cultural imperialism, the doll collectors' world is substantially led by North America. From a doll-collecting perspective the eliding of geographic/national differences may be excused as doll collectors of many nationalities and ethnicities happily see North America as an untroubled focus of desire, an ideal location where new product is freely available and doll collecting for adults is more socially validated. Whilst this may be a naive, under-theorised position, the doll collectors' relative fondness for North America, as leader in the designing and collecting of dolls, co-exists with street protests against globalisation, and emotive claims that George Bush's America has invited retribution from a mistreated Middle East as another and different indication of the opinion of 'ordinary' people that escapes official institutions. The doll particularly identifies doll collectors as a cross section of (generally) non-celebrity men and women and validates their consumption of and affection for fashion.

–3–

When Paris was a Doll: Nineteenth-Century French Couture Dolls

> . . . fashion can only exist and flourish in a particular kind of dramatic setting with knowledgeable fashion performers and spectators . . . the Parisians were 'making it not faking it'. What they were making was the cultural significance of fashion.
>
> Valerie Steele *Paris Fashion* (1999: 135)

If Paris has long been regarded as the site of circulation of and performance of ideas about fashion, then the poupée Parisienne expressed this new visuality and trade in fashionable style in the mid-nineteenth century. If fashion in Second Empire and Third Republic Paris can be defined as a language, then if we avoid discussing the dolls from this era we may be throwing away a quarter or even a third of the pages in the original dictionary. If, as Hollis Clayson and other theorists have argued, the new Paris of the Second Empire was a woman, art and cultural historians have tended to assume that the woman who symbolised Paris was a prostitute. Equally, Paris as woman could be the fantastic, overdressed, over-indulged fashion doll of the Second Empire. By 1885, Emile-Louis Jumeau explicitly named his kid-bodied lady dolls as 'Parisiennes'. He inferred that this name had been in use since 1843, when his father founded his dollmaking business (Cusset 1957: 49, 61–62).

This identification of woman as Paris posited by twentieth-century historians and theorists becomes eerily direct when one contemplates the Antoine Rochard doll, an exceedingly rare porcelain-headed French poupée from c.1867. According to Stuart Holbrook, by 1990 only twelve such dolls were recorded as still existing (1990: 136). Set into her porcelain chest-plate is a series of miniature photographs of the sights of the city of Paris. From a long distance, the photographs appear to hang around the doll's neck like a necklace of cabochon jewels. Even at first glance the doll appears to be a woman of class and culture. In fact, these gleaming spheres are tiny photographs placed under small globes of glass that magnify the tiny scenes so they can be effectively viewed. Such magnified photographs are known as 'Stanhopes' after their British inventor and they were a popular mid-Victorian novelty. The photographs of Paris set into the doll's bust are framed in decorative hand-painted borders of gilt paste and hand-painted enamel. Each doll hitherto documented features a different design in her painting and the doll appears to be wearing an elaborate necklace. They should be dressed with a décolleté evening dress to be seen appropriately. The viewer peers into the white expanse of her cleavage to seek not sexual pleasure, but the look of Napoleon III's new Paris. Antoine Rochard's doll also performs most clearly a duty that Octave Uzanne devolved to all living Parisiennes: to be specifically and effectively fashionable and thus to represent the 'spirit of Paris' (Steele 1999: 9, 137–8, 187). No more literal representation of a female symbolising the city of Paris could be seen than Rochard's doll.

Down the generations the idea that Paris could be a doll rather than a woman has occasionally surfaced. When the Paris correspondent for the *Englishwoman's Domestic Magazine* wished to demonstrate to her readers the abject state into which the city of fashion and pleasure had sunk during the siege and commune of 1871, she could find no clearer metaphor than to report that 'the very doll-shops are devoid of new fashions' (qtd Johnston 1986: 66). The importance of expensive dolls to Paris' reputation was a touchstone to the strange and extreme situation and emphasised the urgent reality of a great crisis in the city. Even today internet guides to 'quaint' or 'authentic' Paris, 'off the beaten track' mention Robert Capia's business selling antique dolls as one of the delights awaiting curious shoppers and overseas visitors in the arcades of Paris (Paris Tourist Office 2003). Capia's merchandise, antique French dolls, still performs the paradigmatic chic that the city has sold for many centuries.

These extraordinary dolls could even stand in for the vanished and legendary women who were Paris in the mid-nineteenth century. The doll, Blondinet Davranches, was found in rural France by an auction house in 1994, apparently in a chateau near Rouen. She had a trousseau of over 150 garments, accessories, personal items and furniture from the Second Empire approximately covering the period of 1862 to 1867. Even her name was recorded in fragile, handwritten notes, whose envelopes bore Napoleon III stamps, sent to the doll in Rouen from Paris by her owner. Through the singular, *unheimlich* discovery of Blondinet and her wardrobe, the French doll is marked with a consumerist promiscuity that is only equalled in recent memory by Imelda Marcos and her similarly inconceivable shoe collection. There sleeping for a century in rural France (as foretold in Perrault's tale) surrounded, naturally, by her wardrobe was the spirit of all those women of the Second Empire, the first, famed consumers of Haute Couture (Marie Antoinette's unfortunate fate is no encouraging advertisement for being a disciple of high fashion) – Pauline Metternich, Cora Pearl, Hortense Schneider, La Paiva and, above all, Eugénie. Considering that Blondinet was found near Rouen, this lady with her extravagant and sumptuous wardrobe could also be linked to the hapless Emma Bovary; however Blondinet was not an aspiring bourgeoise, but a fortunate member of a landed family who wanted for nothing. Blondinet would not die violently for the sake of her incomparable wardrobe and accessories or go into debt over a trousseau for an abortive flight from her home. The women of the Second Empire and their clothes may have departed. In museums and galleries how many dresses can actually be identified as having been worn by any of these early fashion idols? Yet Blondinet's wardrobe remained intact for a hundred years or more until it was finally despoiled in 1994 by that quintessential Second Empire force: the open marketplace.

The development of the Parisian Haute Couture industry in the mid-nineteenth century is familiar to anyone with even a cursory knowledge of the history of fashion. Few people are aware that around the same date a second and parallel industry emerged amongst substantially the same Parisian networks of specialist ateliers and skilled textile workers. This was the luxury doll industry, which specialised in making fine, exclusive and expensively priced dolls. In the period 1850–1880, this luxury trade focussed upon a mature woman in doll form. Throughout the nineteenth century this doll was often named as the Parisienne or the poupée. Other names include Poupée Parisienne and Poupée Peau, referring to the leather bodies used on the dolls. Amongst twentieth-century collectors she was known as the 'French fashion doll', although in recent years collectors have turned to the original nineteenth-century terminology, possibly because doll companies have been manufacturing hard plastic and vinyl dolls also known as 'fashion dolls' for the last half century. The Parisienne was frequently accompanied by a trunk of interchangeable garments and accessories, including hats, shoes and jewellery, all in high fashionable style. The contents of a doll's trousseau frequently extended to furniture and 'homewares'. All these garments and accessories were made by small companies in and around Paris and displayed an extraordinary degree of quality in finish and design. The quality of craft skills is amplified by the small scale of these objects. The packaging of such items was also detailed, stylish and labour-intensive. Engravings were pasted on the lid of coloured cardboard boxes, which were often further embellished with gilt and embossed paper lace. Some French doll accessories were sold in boxes decorated with actual hand-tinted Parisian fashion plates. The advertising copy below the plates advising of the makers and suppliers seems to have been removed, making this packaging for doll clothing and accessories an early example of recycling in the fashion industry.

The doll industry employed much the same publicity and mythmaking strategies as Haute Couture, and from 1850 to 1900 made itself as indispensable to the lifestyle of the wealthy elite of many nations as did Haute Couture fashion. French manufacturers developed another expensive doll, known as the 'bébé'. She was a young girl from a similarly upper-class milieu to the Parisienne, and dressed in perfect examples of the *mode enfantine*. Indications of the original nineteenth-century meaning and usage of the fashionable French doll (which admittedly remain somewhat obscure) place her in an upper-class milieu. A Parisienne auctioned at Sotheby's London in 1999 had a documented provenance as a gift from Queen Victoria to a Scottish nobleman's child when she visited Balmoral for a formal afternoon tea with the Queen c.1876 (Auction Gallery 1999: 16).

Nineteenth-century French dollmakers transformed their trade through the production of fine clothing. Early-nineteenth-century French dolls were sewn into their clothes and it was regarded as a major innovation when Simon-Auguste Brouillet exhibited dolls wearing removable clothing at the 1844 Industrial Exhibition in the Champs-Elysées (Theimer and Theriault 1994: 23). Brouillet presented another innovation: his dolls stood alone without stands (1994: 23). When we are familiar with four decades of boxed fashions by Mattel (and imitators) being freely available for purchase, it is hard to appreciate the possibilities opened up by clothing that was constructed to be independent of the doll, but intended to fit dolls of standardised size. This development is in some ways as conceptually significant as the idea that garments could be produced in standard sizes for humans. It opens up the possibility of handling the garment independently from locating a specific wearer, human or doll. Garments could be made and traded without any wearer being designated or present in the production loop. The wearing was the problem of a person other than the manufacturer, who could produce clothing as a speculation rather than waiting for specific commissions. The simple conceptual leap of making the doll garment no longer dependent upon any specific doll provided the impetus for a vast trade, centred upon Parisian workshops, over the next five decades, in luxury fashionable clothing and accessories for dolls.

The scale or importance of this trade in doll couture should not be underestimated. By 1849, Pierre Jumeau was employing fifty women to make and dress dolls. The quantities of supplies needed in a dollmaking atelier indicate how large these enterprises were. In the Madame Barrois inventory of 1848 (King 2001: 57) the quantities of stock lying in readiness suggest that even at that date the logistics of the Parisian doll industry were not trivial. One finds listings of 1,000 *poupards* (cheap, stiff, unjointed dolls intended to represent swaddled babies), 1,224 varnished papier mâché dolls' heads, 6,164 dolls' heads (of presumably different manufacture or style to the 'papier mâché heads') and 864 dolls' legs. Fabrics for dressing dolls were stocked in equally generous proportions by the Barrois firm, including 1,000 yards of muslin, 110 yards of batiste and 430 yards of tulle, as well as many boxes of flowers and feathers for dolls' millinery. Given that doll-scaled clothing would use less material than human-scaled, the larger number of doll outfits that could be cut from 1,000 yards of muslin indicates the extent of the trade even at this embryonic stage.

Jumeau dolls were commended for their dress alone in the 1840s and 1850s. The Jury of the 1851 Great Exhibition in London stated:

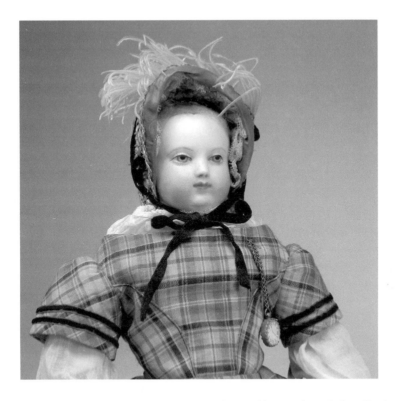

Figure 3.1 Adelaide Huret doll wearing 1850s-era dress and bonnet, formerly in collection of Maurine Popp, image by courtesy of Skinners Auctions, USA.

Prize Medal for dolls dresses. The dolls on which the dresses are displayed present no point worthy of commendation but the dresses themselves are very beautiful productions. Not only are the outer robes accurate representations of the prevailing fashions in ladies' dress but the under garments are in many cases complete facsimiles of those articles of wearing apparel. (qtd King 1983: 18)

If by 1851 French dolls were renowned for their dresses, which perfectly imitated the equally renowned and desired human-scale fashions from Paris, both the French doll trade and the trade in human-scale fashion remained at an early and relatively crude stage. The understanding of the market for fine handwork was still relatively haphazard, as was the branding and identity of the products. The potential for both items and the charisma of the maker to speak in a clear and directed manner to the consumer was hardly developed. Individual products and reputations had not yet acquired the identity of expressing an irresistible lustre and class in themselves. Half a decade before Worth made his breakthroughs in placing and marketing fashion and bringing a new sense of mystique and power to the designer/

supplier, Adelaide Huret had already transformed the ad hoc and anonymous production of dolls by creating a product whose individual style and identity was exclusively associated with her name. Her product was, for a few years, superior to that of her commercial rivals and also unique in the eyes of the buying public, so her product was its own advertisement. These innovations changed the whole identity of the doll. She begot changes in her rivals' dolls as they sought to match the appeal of the Huret product to consumers. Huret's achievement could even be considered to be greater than Worth's, as Huret was socially perhaps less favoured. Though Worth, too, was an outsider as a middle-class Englishman, she as an ageing petit bourgeois spinster was a person specifically unfavoured in French discourses of public life and public culture. It is curious that the impetus to reform the French garment trade came so definitely from 'outsiders', especially if one recalls that Worth's original partner and financial backer was a Swedish colleague, Otto Bobergh. Adelaide Huret was an unmarried daughter of a prosperous merchant family. At thirty-seven, when she patented her dolls, she was no longer considered young. As an unmarried woman she would be regarded as a 'failure' in petit bourgeois and bourgeois households. As an ageing spinster Adelaide Huret would – in the normal course of events – be considered irrelevant and invisible by the society around her. Yet she created a significant artform, brought in much foreign capital to France and made a tangible contribution to quantifying the elusive idea of 'French style' in an international marketplace through developing and putting into practice the ambition to design a more beauti- ful doll.

The transformations that Huret made in the marketing of luxury consumer goods in Paris survive into the present day. Likewise her innovations survive in a cheapened format in every 'pink aisle' of discount stores like K-Mart and toy shop chains like Toys 'R' Us: the provisioning of dolls with ready-made wardrobes and accessories. Her achievement is even more unusual when one considers the position from which she started. Contemporary readers can appreciate the com- plexity of Adelaide Huret's starting point and innovative approach due to François Theimer translating and publishing details of her patent application. By her own admission, Huret was spurred onto doll designing by the poor appearance of the dolls currently being sold in France. 'The deformed shapes of dolls found in shops today must have made many people think that an improvement is possible.' She adds 'what's more its roughly designed shape in no way suits it for dressing up, almost completely discouraging the decorator' (qtd Theimer 1997: 85). Yet it was not only the law of the eye that Huret sought to address, she was also motivated by a maternalist concern to anticipate the needs of the child, reinforcing Formanek- Brunell's identification of professional commercial dollmaking as a site which domestic feminist values could be asserted and put into practice (1993: 3). In Huret's concern for the 'justness' of the doll to the perceived needs of the well-adjusted child, in a well-regulated home, we can see the political and social dimension of domestic feminist aspirations.

> An articulated body, capable of imitating basic human movements and whose shape, without being over perfect for a child's toy, nevertheless is close enough to reality to please the eye – such an idea must have gone through the heads of all those in contact with the sorry examples available at present . . . Even [the jointed layfigure] belonging to the painter, though cleverly made is equally unsuitable as a child's plaything. (Adelaide Huret qtd Theimer 1997: 85)

Where Huret's maternalist sentiments are most clearly articulated is in the protective concern that just as Caesar's things must be rendered unto Caesar and God's unto God, so should the child play only with that which is relevant to her. Thus Huret is concerned to identify what is appropriate to the child and demarcate the child's things from pollution by that which is appropriate to the adult. Therefore Huret identifies childhood as a vulnerable state, easily corrupted or distorted by contact with the adult world. Many of the anxieties that are raised around Barbie are those of contagion and confusion: she introduces adult concepts into a child's world and educates girls to be materialistic and vapid, the least socially useful of women. Yet this anxiety about the permeable borders between the adult and the child arises a century earlier than Barbie, through the dolls of Adelaide Huret. If Huret saw a deeply seriously pedagogical function for her dolls as training girls in womanly duties, the industry that rapidly developed in the wake of her innovative dollmaking became the site for conspicuous consumption and brought the celebration of rituals and dress of the high society woman into the milieu of childhood. Huret herself condoned this change of direction when her original intention of educating young girls proved unworkable.

> The lady-inventor's original idea was that the dolls, which she sold virtually naked, should be clothed by the child owner. However, little girls' fingers are sometimes clumsy and the busy mothers called to help with the sewing had other things to do. The call went out for ready-made clothing . . . and so it is now seamstresses, furriers, shoemakers, fine woodworkers and a whole range of other occupations are engaged in work related to this new industry which the Huret doll created and which in its turn gives rise to new specialists . . . Around the Rue de Choiseul a number of dolls' clothes makers have set up their workshops, and made their fortune several times over. (Henri Nicolle c.1867 qtd Theimer 1997: 88)

Huret herself must have condoned the luxury production standards attained by the range of dolls, clothes and accessories marketed under her name, as well as the high prices. Documentation does not speak of her introducing a budget or accessible model, so the appeal of the gaze won over the instructional value and the prudent guardianship of the unprotected child's interests. Huret became renowned as the founder of the luxury Parisian doll industry, not as a reformer of childhood playthings. At the time of the 1867 Paris exhibition, in a long discussion of Huret's dolls, French Journalist Henri Nicolle stated 'the Huret dolls have created a whole new industry in the field of luxury dolls and have rightly earned a place in toy history' (qtd Theimer 1997: 87).

The innovation of Huret's dolls runs beyond high fashion. They are very early examples of plastic toys. Her doll's body was not sewn from cloth or leather; she chose a pliable moulding material, gutta-percha, for her doll bodies. As each part of her jointed doll had to be produced in separately tooled moulds, the expense of producing extra moulds and retooling for a size range prevented her from producing the dolls in a greater size range. Gutta-percha is derived (like rubber and latex) from the sap of a Malaysian tree. Though superseded by many other substances, gutta-percha is recognised as being amongst the earliest commercially viable plastic compounds. Huret's choice of body material further demonstrates her complex positioning of her dolls. The novelty and relative unfamiliarity of this substance to the feminine domestic world must not be underestimated. Adelaide Huret's dolls were, in effect, a smash-and-grab raid upon science and technology from the worlds of creative arts, high fashion and domestic feminism.

Even today, in Western society, the fields of science and technology still guard not only the esteem that their masculine identity guarantees, but their privileged status in the eyes of government, educational and economic bodies, against the relatively undervalued creative vocations. Elsa Schiaparelli is routinely commended by historians of dress for her breadth of intellect, which permitted collaboration in the 1930s not only with Surrealist artists, but with manufacturers of synthetic fabrics and substances, to expand the range of possibilities for fashion. In marketing an early and successful plastic-polymer-bodied doll and in developing a luxury industry and mystique around her name, Adelaide Huret seems to have consistently paralleled the mindset of acknowledged fashion innovators, including Schiaparelli as well as Worth. The use of plastic for children's toys is now so widespread as to be taken for granted and obscure Huret's achievements, but there could be no Toys 'R' Us, no injection moulding plants on upper stories of Hong Kong high rises or in polluted industrial estates in China, no legions of Pedigree, Regal, Ideal or Mattel dolls in their collective billions without such early successful examples of plastic technology as the Huret doll. That gutta-percha would, in the long run, prove to be fragile, and many Huret-designed porcelain heads ended up being fitted to replacement bodies, did not prevent this plastic-bodied doll being sold for at least seventeen years. Only changes of ownership in the company took the Huret doll off the market, not customer dissatisfaction.

If the Second Empire was the era in which Haussmann and Worth emerged to become household names, it was also the era of the no less spectacular and transformative rise of Adelaide Huret and her dolls. Huret's dolls were as modern and finely wrought as the creations of Worth and Haussmann. As with Worth in dress and Haussmann in city planning, Huret established a position from which the experience of modernity could never retreat nor degenerate. If Worth and Haussmann could be paired in metaphor as symbol/mirror of each other's achievement, Huret's dolls share this grand vision – the faith in the mutability of matter, and triumph of style and construction, the unification provided by the eye and mind of the designer. If Haussmann constructed a city of sweeping, united direction and a visually cohesive style, from the foetid alleys and crumbling buildings of *le veille Paris*, then the beautiful Huret poupée with her superbly constructed garments and her pretty but naturalistic face likewise swept aside and improved upon the often ramshackle doll norms of yesteryear.

Certainly, for the Jumeau company, the analogy between the development of the city of Paris, with its transformed public life and amenity, and the development of a new, sophisticated improved format of doll, was direct. The development of the doll trade was a positivist one, in line with the Third Republic's belief in science, system and order. That the rapid development of the French doll trade can be fairly attributed to the direct initiative of one woman, Adelaide Huret (although of course she would not be acknowledged in the publication promoting a major male-directed dollmaking enterprise) is all the more remarkable. Likewise remarkable is how Cusset's train of argument so closely prefigures later twentieth-century academic theory around the modernity of Paris, especially the sense of transformation and the virtu ascribed to the cleansing/salvation/rebirthing of the city.

Time marches on and new inventions were everywhere surprising the world, which could hardly believe its eyes. After the railroads there were telegrams, then sewing machines and a host of innovations which will make this period renowned.

The old shops full of dust were demolished wholesale, and on their ruins arose elegant and spacious new ones full of light and luxuriously appointed. In place of smoky oil lamps gas flared in opalescent globes, windows sparkled to attract the passers by and the old people, astonished, wondered by what wave of the fairy wand all these miracles have taken place. The whole world was turned upside down and in no time all the antiquities disappeared and their place taken by novelty and progress.

Today, scarcely 30 years after this industrial revolution, it is only very seldom, in some small hidden corner of the capital that one finds a 'boutique' of our parents' time to serve as a reminder of what we all were like.

It is at this period that the two Jumeau sons wanted to follow the new ideas. (Cusset 1957: 63–6)

Notice, for Cusset and Jumeau, retailing and the public face of the shop are the chief indicators for calibrating urban growth and development.

Other women would copy Huret's ideas. Leontine Rohmer would prove to be particularly irksome to Huret, as Schiaparelli was to Chanel. Huret regarded Rohmer's dolls as copies. In 1861, the two women went into court over plagiarisms and patent infringements. Huret was spurred on to further develop wrist and neck jointings of her dolls (Theimer 1997: 87). Poor Leontine Rohmer has been cast in later historians' accounts as the knock-off queen of the Parisian doll trade, the Joan Crawford 'bitch', the warped and jealous Salieri, who could not claim true creative independence. It is even claimed that Rohmer acquired a public award, the bronze medal at the 1867 Paris exhibition, through (unspecified) underhand means (Theimer and Theriault 1994: 61). However, many of Rohmer's dolls survive from the 1850s onwards, suggesting that her product found willing buyers. They are well produced and stylishly dressed and certainly do not deserve their recent bad press. In 1971 John Noble, at least, rightfully described a Rohmer doll as a 'superb' example, with an 'alert and distinctive' face (Noble 1971: 112–13).

Jenny Béreux was originally a dressmaker employed by Huret, but she moved out to establish a business under her own name using part of the premises of her parents' perfume business. At the time of the 1867 exhibition, Béreux was regarded as 'the founder of the speciality of making garments for dolls, a field which has undergone unbelievable expansion since she invented it' as the exhibition Jury stated (Theriault 1994: 9). Béreux was criticised at the 1862 London Exhibition for the extreme standards of luxury and the high costs of the dolls' dresses that she sold and exhibited (Theimer and Theriault 1994: 50). This negative reaction to Béreux's designs directly echoes the critiques directed at Barbie, suggesting, as do various critiques of fashionable dolls throughout the nineteenth and early-twentieth centuries that the anxieties raised by fashion dolls are paradigmatic and long-standing and do not only address Barbie as a singular and inappropriate incursion of transnational capitalism into a child's life.

Madame Lavallée-Peronne founded a luxury magazine, *La Poupée Modèle*, in 1863, which promoted Parisian dolls and their fashions. As well as those of the founder's maison, *La Poupée Modèle* also advertised dolls by other major companies. *La Poupée Modèle* also inspired trade rivals entitled *La Poupée* and *Gazette de la Poupée* (King 1983: 26). All of these magazines frequently advertised social activities for girls and their dolls taking place at dollmakers' ateliers. They presented dolls, including those by Béreux and Jumeau, in coloured plates, engraved and lithographed, of the latest designs with inscriptions identifying the inventors and suppliers, just like the adult fashion magazines. Doll play in Napoleon III's Paris was an apprenticeship for future social responsibility and roles. By the early-1900s, *La Poupée Modèle* was a sister publication to a mainstream French fashion magazine, *Le Journal des Demoiselles*, according to its cover, and the two publications seem to have been linked even in the early-1860s. *Le Journal des Demoiselles* apparently absorbed another major title, *Le Petit Courier des*

Dames, and featured work by renowned artists such as Laure Noel. *La Poupée Modèle* could boast credible fashion connections.

The structure of the Second Empire and Third Republic Parisian doll trade was complex. The manufacturers were dependent upon one another and traded with one another. These exact patterns of trade and supply are hard to track, but we can outline some of the interdependent loops through which dolls were marketed. Some dollmakers such as Steiner sold only to other wholesalers and retailers. Huret both made and sold dolls. The Jumeau firm would later do likewise, although at first it sold only to wholesalers. During the 1850s and 1860s Pierre Jumeau sold on dolls by other makers, including Steiner, and fine imported wax dolls from British manufacturers. English wax dolls had a following amongst Parisian consumers and were considered chic and exclusive. Manufacturers of porcelain heads sold to other dollmakers, as well as producing product under their own names. Some firms assembled dolls with heads bought from other manufacturers. Other firms never made or assembled dolls but dressed and accessorised dolls purchased from other makers. Dress or accessory items were made in independent ateliers and supplied to other firms assembling dolls. Some companies sold doll clothes and accessories direct to the public and others did not produce dolls but sold luxury dolls made by other hands to customers off the street. Those who sold dolls to the public usually labelled them with the name of their house, and the product of many of these firms can be identified today: Simonne, Au Paradis des Enfants, Aux Rêves des Enfants, Lavallée-Peronne, A L'Enfant Sage, Au Nain Bleu, Au Nain Jaun, Perreaux, A La Poupée de Nuremberg, Au Bengali, Au Calife de Bagdad, Aux Bébés Sages, Aux Enfants Sages are some of the names of luxury doll and toy shops in Paris found printed on labels on the bodies of poupées and bébés from the 1860s onwards. The number of different firms indicates the scale of the trade. Many of them were run by women. Of this list Au Nain Bleu is still trading in Paris. According to Florence Theriault, Au Nain Bleu had their own workshops for 'designing and making doll's trousseaux and presentations. It was said that the entire court of Napoleon III shopped for toys at the store' (Theriault 1998: 44).

The poupée was also sold by speciality stores for fashion, accessories and household linen. A box for a Jumeau poupée carries a label for a Biarritz store specialising modern and antique in lace, especially of Spanish origin (Theimer and Theriault 1994: 226). This combination of selling both dolls and fashion garments under the same roof in a small business would seem impossible by today's marketing conventions, although deploying the Barbie doll for publicity purposes and licensing revenue does bring fashion and the doll in greater contact in the present day. The Parisian stores specialising in selling expensive dolls modelled themselves on luxury emporiums already selling novelties and accessories in Paris. The doll trade was developed through an understanding of this exclusive level of retailing. Adelaide Huret's family were locksmiths and makers of iron furniture.

Their clients included the French royal family and the court after the restoration of the Bourbon monarchy, and the Hurets held warrants as court suppliers. Leon Casimir Bru's dolls were dressed by his wife, a professional seamstress, who was the daughter of a master tailor. As said above, Jenny Béreux had worked as a dressmaker for Adelaide Huret. That she then began selling doll couture from a corner of her parents' perfumery (Theriault 1994: 9) is another link to luxury industries in Paris.

If, as Valerie Steele has noted, the milliners working at the luxury end of the trade regarded themselves as the aristocrats of the working class, artists in their own right (Steele 1999: 70–72), then the Parisian families working in these substantial household-based doll ateliers may also have seen themselves as similarly independent, as artists, rather than as workers. Certainly the Jumeau family made an astonishing transition from artisans to landed gentry on the profits of selling dolls. Emile-Louis Jumeau and his family came to live the lifestyle which their dolls were intended to represent, in a manner more expected from their clients. Early-twentieth-century photographs show that the Jumeaus retained the trappings of an elegant country life after selling off their doll company (Theimer and Theriault 1994: 111–12, 185–9). François Gaultier, who supplied porcelain heads to many smaller ateliers, served as Mayor in the village of St Maurice outside Paris from 1886 to 1892 (Seeley 1992: 79), suggesting that, like Jumeau, he was a person of status and solidity in the community.

The catalogue-album published in 1994 for the auction of the wardrobe of Blondinet Davranches is the best indication of the parameters of the fashionable French nineteenth-century doll's world (Theriault 1994). Her trousseau included not only clothes and accessories but also many three-dimensional objects, including the gilded, cast-iron doll furniture made by the Huret firm, which was an exact doll-sized replica of the adult-sized iron furniture marketed by the Huret family. There were two hammocks, one in a box from the Au Calife de Bagdad store in Paris, a folding ebony and black velvet campaign chair and even miniature hand-forged fire irons, the latter attributed to Huret. In the detailed documentation of each tiny item in the surviving trousseau can one see the completeness of the emulation of the world of the fashionable beauty of good family (for Blondinet's aristocratic provenance is an indication of the intended market), and also the rococo folly and excess of replicating a fashionable lady and her wardrobe in miniature. The bespoke customising extends even to her initials 'B' for Blondinet on such items as her jewellery and her notepaper. In the folly of this quest to replicate in dead perfection, the world of the living, one can discern the conceptual strength of fashion, its urges and its capacity to create objects of extraordinary singularity, which, when analysed, make little sense, yet on their own terms carry a consummate conviction. Blondinet documents the rigid world of her owner, with a sense of contextual richness that 'period' films lack. The detail of Blondinet's world – now scattered – also suggests how difficult it is for the museum, collector or production designer to actually pinpoint the details of, to replicate, another period. What stylist or designer dressing a play or film would be literate in the range of multiple veils, collars, lappets, hairnets, snoods, lace net and tatted stoles, undersleeves and engageantes that are included with the expected crinoline dresses, shoes, gloves, capes and hats? How could a tripper from a later era do anything other than assemble pastiches of this range of subtly differentiated garments? The outsider, the viewer from another time, can only hope to reassemble fragments of the original meanings and phrases.

Blondinet's world in turn horrifies and enchants. Her world horrifies to the extent that it invokes a neo-Marxist awareness of class and inequality. Blondinet's world may be equally horrifying in feminist terms. From the accessories we can tell much about the assumed character and occupations of Blondinet (and the culture that she taught). She was a Catholic, for she owns a turquoise-studded crucifix and her reticule holds a book, with an ivory cover, entitled *Messe*. She owns no other books, but is well supplied with a writing portfolio, sealing wax and seals, a chair and table, a writing stand with ink bottles, pencils and a pen. No doubt she wrote a journal, kept family members informed of various developments and news and supervised the menus, if not the daily accounts. As one would expect, Blondinet has a fine sewing companion, with tiny gold scissors, ivory tools, tiny bone thimble, thread and pieces of tatting. The myriad dresses recall how upper-class French women's lives were so exquisitely regimented, each dress suitable for different activities throughout the day. Women visiting the Second Empire court at the Chateau of Compiègne were expected to bring a change of dress in styles appropriate to every social occasion from the hunt to the ball, and never appear in the same garment twice (E.A. Coleman 1989: 14; Dolan 1994: 22; Steele 1999: 140–41). Blondinet's now-scattered dresses tell the story of a ritualised, ordered life in which women – well regulated and behaved – could be read to provide signs of social order and cohesion. The life that the real woman lived hardly allowed any self-expression or exploration. It could even be performed as effectively by dolls as women; no wonder that for many male thinkers since the enlightenment, the idea of the doll and the woman were inextricably intertwined (Peers 1997: 72–6). Blondinet and her legions of sister Parisiennes are the voices, the lives that are obliterated by the avant-garde.

Translated into a doll form, removed from her round of pietistic, class and social obligations, the world of the nineteenth-century French gentry woman, always more ritualised, ordered and surveilled than that of her English contemporaries, begins to have a charm of its own. Thus can Blondinet's trousseau enchant as well as horrify. Through the wardrobe of the doll we can appreciate the sensuous vividness and diversity of the material textures and forms of the upper-class Frenchwoman's life, the perfection of each finely shaped and organised detail. We can reclaim and applaud the skills inherent in the delicate, yet fantastic, bonnets in fragile chiffon and silk tulle over miniature hand-wrought wire frames, trimmed with tiny frills. Do we demand that these objects express a social and historical responsibility – in which they fail – because they are predominantly by women or used in a female realm?

Certainly in Constance Eileen King's account of Jumeau dolls (King 1983: 9) the regulation of female life amongst the nineteenth-century French aristocracy and bourgeoisie becomes for her an almost racist sign of the Otherness, the strangeness, of the French and, by implication, the naturalness and normality of British values. Cogently, she identifies that the extraordinary French dolls of the nineteenth century, whilst loved internationally when made, had a special relationship to the legal and social position of 'respectable' women in France at the period (1983: 10). For outsiders they had a different but no less *French* identity. Rather than speaking of female behaviour and self-management's responsibility to family and class, for foreigners the Parisian doll was a sign of fashion itself, 'and if the young of America or Bavaria found them quite unlike the women they saw around them, this, in a way, added to their allure as products of that fashionable, fast city Paris' (1983: 10). It is, however, too easy to see this role played by French women only in terms of its reductive nature as indicated by King's account. Whilst, ironically, women's agency was so reduced that their functions in guarding and vouchsafing family assets could be as well played by a doll, surely the message of Offenbach's 1881 opera the *Tales of Hoffman* (Peers 1997: 74), Edith Wharton's short story *Madame de Treymes*, 1906, indicates the seriousness of the familial responsibilities entrusted to women in propertied families in France. Wharton emphasises the complex role women played on behalf of a family's reputation and general financial and dynastic interests (Wharton 1995).[1]

Yet the trousseau of Blondinet Davranches tells not only a story of class exploitation and difference. Blondinet's luxurious clothes speak not of indigent criminal underclasses, but of those women, prudent and diligent, as la Fontaine's ant, who managed these Parisian ateliers, who grew up in families literate in the tradition of servicing and supplying aristocratic customers and who gained a sense of self-worth from having supplied the very best to their exclusive clientele. These women were unsung artists, able to devise and flawlessly execute these confections to grace the wardrobes of Blondinet and the thousands – even millions – of lady dolls produced in Paris between 1850 and 1900, so many of which still survive. The report of the 1855 Paris exhibition praised Pierre Jumeau's senior worker, Mademoiselle Delphine Floss:

> Maker of dolls for five years, intelligent and adroit, she has contributed greatly to the success of the firm by the creation of new models and by the care which she brings to the execution of orders. Her conduct is exemplary. She maintains by her work her aged mother and three young children. (qtd King 1983: 22)

Whereas most of the once-admired female names of nineteenth-century French fashion have disappeared into limbo (Steele 1991: 23), some doll couturiers can be recalled through their firmly labelled product, even if, apart from Huret, it is currently hard to read a house style from company to company, as there has been very little analysis and cataloguing of the contents of public and private collections. As well as items from Huret, three dresses in Blondinet's trousseau bear labels of Jenny Béreux.

If adult-sized couture is accepted as effective gallery fare on formal grounds of orchestration of colour, of playing with texture and form, of executive and conceptual skill, then these doll-sized couture dresses deserve more attention in public institutions. Moreover the women who made and/or devised these miniature dresses deserve acknowledgement as artists and creators. Everything in the trousseau of Blondinet Davranches – if we take it as an exemplar – invokes admiration for the skill of these Parisian women as designers, as entrepreneurs and – both they themselves and their employees – as seamstresses and executants. These dresses have the seriousness of authentic couture and its turn of emphatic statement. Often the dresses will encompass *le mot juste* of a stylish exaggeration to catch the eye: an overly long sash, a contrasting trim, a focal point of decoration, a fastening or a button. There is crisp precision in the sewing and application of soutache braiding in intricate patterns and various colourways. There is the fine handling of delicate laces and beadwork, the fantasy of millinery constructions and precision of cut in the dresses and coats. The dress sold as lot forty-four shows decisiveness and authority in the handling of a bright plaid, matched with faultless placing of the velvet banding. Even the seemingly trivial and ordinary pieces in the trousseau lack nothing. Each translucent muslin undersleeve or blouse is meticulously tucked; each collar is individually shaped and decorated; no two are the same, and every set of underwear is trimmed in a different style, yet all conform to an overriding pattern of outline and format of early-1860s daywear. A series of matching petticoats and drawers shows a wide variety of white-on-white techniques, and the waistbands are differently cut on each set. Couture garments are widely renowned for the care taken over hidden details, and Blondinet's trousseau fully meets the exacting and ideal standards of couture in this respect.

Adelaide Huret employed the finest available standards of work for items that were supposedly trivial, and carried elite style down to the smallest detail and scale. Ironically, as physical objects, Huret's dolls themselves were not imitated. As discussed she only had one basic set of head and body moulds, so her dolls were always one size: eighteen inches high. Her use of the polymer gutta-percha to make a body that was superior to the stuffed leather bodies was generally not followed except by some makers in producing an alternative to the leather body. Leontine Rohmer would experiment with lightweight metal bodies (again a female producing a hard, supposedly 'masculine', doll body!). The Gesland firm presented a doll with wool padding and a knitted jersey covering over a metal armature (males working with softly contoured dolls). In 1867 Madame Clement patented a hollow pressed-leather body. However the majority of Parisiennes would retain the leather body with gusset joints first used in the 1830s with papier mâché heads. By the 1860s, this body had already been pronounced as superseded by Huret's advocates, and as the cause of incurable 'wasting disease' amongst young doll ladies once their seams split (Nicolle qtd Theimer 1997: 88). Note the facetious use of the language of disease and weakness associated with young women to describe splitting seams in a sewn leather body. Collectors are familiar with this fault. The faces of Huret's dolls were not so frequently imitated. They were more jowly than the standard face favoured by dollmakers in Paris, which was a long, slim face with inset glass eyes (slightly large in proportion to the face), and a finely modelled mouth. There are some exceptions to this rule. Jumeau's lady dolls from 1880 onwards increasingly shared the moulds of his child dolls, and featured eyes that became over life-size, prefiguring the Japanese anime representations of the face, and tipping the doll towards a surrealistic and artificial stylisation.

The French doll was inspired by the features of the Empress Eugénie, who was so closely associated with the development of the French fashion trade. The doll's face outlived the reign of the empress, being as popular in the Third Republic as it was during the Second Empire. Theimer notes that the beautiful Eugénie was 'beloved, revered' amongst the French populace (1991: 20). Eugénie made a crucial contribution not only to the development of the fashion trade but also to modern mass-media imaging of women. She is perhaps an early indication of the imbricated investment of high fashion and the media in exceptional women. Diana, Marilyn and Madonna can all be traced back to Eugénie as popular sign of 'beauty'. Therese Dolan suggests that Eugénie was regarded as a trendsetter who made styles as much as did named designers (1994: 22). Her role as inspiration for dolls' faces indicates that dolls have played a part in spinning the legends of these singular women. Due to photography, she was the first internationally beloved supermodel. Photographs and the paintings of Winterhalter made Eugénie's reputation. For her contemporaries, she was particularly fascinating amongst European royalty, as the soupçon of commonness in her background made her more accessible. She was a mere countess. 'Real' princesses had refused the hand of Napoleon III or as in the case of the Princess Hohenlohe her family had refused him on her behalf to her great distress, for marriage was too important an alliance to be left to young, untested girls. Simultaneously Eugénie's status as wife, empress and strong Catholic believer made her more ethereal than many of the venal and mercenary women in Napoleon III's life; although Eugénie herself was also read as a venal manipulator indistinguishable from the other ambitious and sexually devious women around the emperor.

Art historian Therese Dolan indicates that not only a generalised concept of the 'prostitute' haunted avant-garde French imaging of women in the 1860s, but pictures, cartoons and writing were laced with specific anxieties about Eugénie's de facto political interference (1997: 611–29). Not only did the sophisticated assume Eugénie had 'favourites', because, of course, all women when in positions of social and political independence were sexually predatory, but they believed that such favourites and lovers were placed in politically influential positions (Dolan 1994: 24–5). Now that a greater range of sexual freedoms are publicly acceptable amongst women, popular historians have once again elevated Eugénie as Queen of the Whores (Rees 2003: 7–8), the symbolic role that Dolan believes informed Manet's *Olympia*. In some ways, all the possible symbols of Napoleon III's regime seem to converge: new city, luxurious shops, high fashion, prostitutes, dolls and Eugénie.

Collectors have long claimed that various dolls were portraits of Eugénie, for example Rachel Field, an American children's author of great renown in the interwar years, owned a Parisienne whom she named 'Empress Eugénie'. The 'empress' featured in photographs published in *Child Life* magazine, 1935 (Baker 1986: 102, 106). François Theimer states that the Bru company definitely intended the faces of their poupées to be portraits of Eugénie (1991: 20). Elsewhere he suggests that the empress provided an inspiration to French dollmakers generally (Theimer and Theriault 1994: 54). The Barrois company also sculpted a 'Eugénie' face. In some doll faces the resemblance to Eugénie was more generic than portrait-like, but overall one can point to the strongly oval face, the elongated nose, the defined lips and a strongly frontal orientation of the facial features as elements that Parisienne dolls hold in common with photographs as well as artistic representations of Eugénie.

The Parisiennes or poupées were popular from the 1850s to the 1890s, although, through dress and other styling elements, one can suggest that the greatest period of popularity for the dolls appears to be from the later-1860s to the early-1880s. Advertisements for Au Paradis des Enfants around the early-1860s indicate that the high standard of production in Blondinet Davranches' trousseau was the norm not the exception. The shop distributed tiny *carte de visites* bearing photographs of dolls in fashionable ensembles, thus placing dolls in the same system of public visibility as actresses, queens and fashionable beauties. These photographs were collected into small albums and Mario Tosa regards these Au Paradis des Enfants albums as prefiguring the Barbie doll booklets of the early-1960s (1998: 10), again indicating how Mattel's supposedly unique innovations replicate stratagems of French dollmakers a century earlier.

Au Paradis des Enfants presented a dressed doll wearing a meticulous copy of a cashmere shawl, as found in the trousseau of Blondinet Davranches, with intricate patterned repeat weaving. Experienced handweavers in wool were obviously

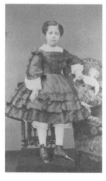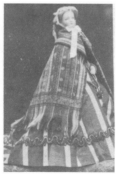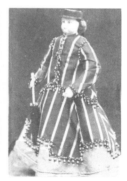

Figure 3.2 Left to right: *carte de visite* of child with doll c.1860 by Pierre Petit, 31 Place Cadet Paris; two *cartes de visites* with inscription verso 'Au Paradis des Enfants. Maison Perreau Fils. Jouets Magazin le plus vaste de Paris 156, rue de Rivoli et 1, rue du Louvre.

being commissioned to produce these items in small scale. In this early photograph (see Figure 3.2, middle doll), the shawl is worn in the manner of a fashionable burnous over a very wide crinoline skirt of the early-1860s. Another doll in original dress from the early-1860s is illustrated by John Noble (1971: 118). She wears a silk walking dress and a floral bonnet, indicating again that by c.1860 the Parisienne had already developed into her characteristic format, as she has a bisque head rather than glazed china. Many dolls can be found in the princess lines and flaring skirts of the later 1860s. Another photographic advertisement, from Au Paradis des Enfants (see Figure 3.2, doll on right), indicates a doll in a slightly later dress of two parts with a flaring striped jacket – reflecting Worth's concern in the later-1860s with avoiding the use of seam line between skirt and bodice – and the narrower skirts of about c.1867. It is trimmed with an elaborate braid of silk-wrapped beads, more typical of upholstery decoration. She wears a 'porkpie' hat and a large chignon, typical of this slightly later period. Mario Tosa illustrates further photographs from the series of Au Paradis des Enfants advertisements, including a male doll dressed as a French officer, with plumed helmet and epaulettes, a doll in early-1860s evening dress and a later 1860s doll in a short-skirted walking dress (1998: 11). The variety and detail of these ensembles documented in Au Paradis des Enfants publicity surpasses the oeuvre of surviving dolls. The crinoline evening dress in the photograph illustrated by Tosa is particularly impressive.

The styles worn most frequently by Parisiennes and poupées date from the 1870s, especially the heavily draped bustle styles of the early years of this decade. The intricate cutting and styling of 1870s high fashion, with its elaborate draping and myriad trimmings, such as ruching and box pleating and flouncing in self or contrasting colours, is a challenge easily met by French dollmakers and doll

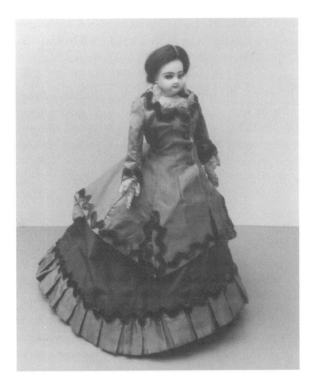

Figure 3.3 Parisienne by Jumeau wearing original brown taffeta and velvet demi-evening dress by Ernestine Jumeau, early- to mid-1880s.

couturiers of the era. Detailing at cuffs and necklines is reproduced with particular fidelity, despite the complexities demanded by double or even triple layers of trimmings, ruching, banding, laces, cording, rouleaux, etc. A Jumeau doll from the early- to mid-1880s in a private collection documents the eclipse of the bustle c.1880, although the slightly flaring cut of the dress would perhaps be a small exaggeration for the sake of aesthetics to give the doll more presence (see Figure 3.3). The two tones of brown taffeta belong, as anyone who has handled a museum collection of nineteenth-century dresses would know, to the familiar colour palette of the period from green greys, through to taupes, to chocolate browns to beige and silver grey. In other contexts, these colours would be seen as inexpressibly dowdy, yet they were handled with much discrimination in early-1880s fashion and contrast with the riot of aniline colours favoured in the previous two decades. The Powerhouse Museum, Sydney holds a particularly fine 1880s Parisienne with an Au Nain Bleu label. Her green dress in plain and floral-patterned silk features multiple panels of smocking, a favourite decorative technique in this era. A number of Jumeau Parisiennes document the heavily draped fashions of the mid-1880s, including the sparkling jet and beaded trims characteristic of the period. Even though the company did not recommend them and was renowned for its children's fashions, Ernestine Jumeau, who designed and approved of the dolls' outfits, effectively mirrored adult fashions throughout the decade.

As well as townwear and eveningwear, many Parisiennes wear printed cotton or crisp white muslin, with broad-brimmed hats, appropriate attire for summer on the family estate. Both Parisiennes and earlier papier mâché French dolls were frequently dressed as nuns. The meticulous detail with which the frequently archaic underclothing and accessories of French religious dress is recreated provides useful records for the costume historian. Sometimes a Parisienne dressed as a nun may be furnished with a suitable trousseau. Her garments could include fine dresses from the world that she renounced for her vow of poverty – indicating her genteel status before she took Holy Orders – an elaborate, fashionable white ensemble for her Dedication, a novice's uniform and a full habit. Some Parisiennes wear provincial and regional dress, of varying degrees of authenticity as decorative souvenirs and ornaments or gentrified fancy-dress interpretations of picturesque rural clothing. Eighteenth-century fashions were also frequently interpreted by French doll-makers, including pastoral characters and aristocrats. Other dolls replicate racial stereotypes long popular with both the *juste milieu* and avant-garde of French artists: seductive odalisques in veils and spangled gauzes, gypsies in hot-coloured satins and gold ornaments, señoritas, geishas, Chinese concubines with embroidered lotus shoes, mulattos in bright checked turbans, skirts and off-the-shoulder blouses. Of all the female chimeras who haunt nineteenth-century art, only the ballet dancer seems absent.[2] Some Parisiennes had strongly patriotic meanings including post-1870 dolls in Alsatian dress, dolls dressed as *vivandières* in the colours of French regiments or as St Geneviéve, the patron saint of Paris. Many of these fancy dolls were 'despised' by collectors throughout the twentieth century, who re-dressed them in pastiches of nineteenth-century town clothes.

French artists portray dolls so accurately that the slimmer Parisienne or poupée of the 1860s or 1870s can be distinguished from the chubbier bébé or child doll of the 1880s. Renoir portrays French dolls as part of a fashionable *mise en scène*. In *Mother and Children*, (c.1876–78. Oil on canvas. Frick collection) the image of the fashionable Parisienne is replicated three times in decreasing scale, from the lady to her daughters, to the child holding a fashion doll. The mother and the Parisienne doll wear virtually the same styles, a dark: possibly velvet, jacket with a bow at the neck. This work places the doll in the context of fashionable display in a public park. Behind the main group there are other fashionable strollers and nursemaids employed by prosperous families. Renoir indicates the soft stuffed kid body of the doll in its slightly lax bearing. Conversely, in *Children's Afternoon at Wargemont* (1884. Oil on canvas. Nationalgalerie, Berlin) he indicates a composition-bodied bébé, able to sit upright, distinguished by its heavier and more substantial materiality, large feet and hands. The elastic-strung bébé could assume a greater variety of attitudes and has a more solid bearing. In both paintings he places the doll amongst the stylish bourgeoisie. In the *Children's Afternoon*, Renoir painted the children of a colleague and patron. By placing the doll in this continuum of style, Renoir gives an indication of how the French doll was used and understood.

Marriage in nineteenth-century-upper class French society was not a romantic but a contractual relation. Mutual desire and personal charm played little part in brokering alliances. Therefore, as Valerie Steele suggests, wealthy and respectable young girls in Paris were expected to be neither 'sexually attractive' nor adept in 'lively' conversation. A beautiful, gifted wife and mother was not only a suave and reliable performer on social occasions, but 'her daughter's best advertisement, as well as the guardian of her sexual innocence'. The mother was also 'supposed to be charming' to her daughter's fiancé 'as a kind of promise of what the daughter would become' (Steele 1999: 156). In the circuitousness of the image of fashionable beauty from doll to child to mother to doll seen in Renoir's *Mother and Children*, it is possible that just as the mother provides guidance and instruction from above to the child, as well as an imprimatur to those wishing to ally themselves to the silent daughter, so, too, the doll as fashionable woman in the arms of a girl is another indication that the child is being surrounded by the best of exemplars in training her to her social and personal obligations.

As part of the marketing of style in Paris dolls feature in fashion plates. Artists sometimes place the doll in the hands of children, sometimes in the hands of adults. A twentieth-century audience would expect the doll to be firmly indicated as belonging in the world of children, as she is in some fashion plates where the child is either nursing her or otherwise playing with her. In one plate, c.1860, reproduced by John Noble (1971: 119), the adult hands the doll to a child, indicating the doll's pedagogical function within wealthy women's mission of display. In an 1857 French plate by Laure Noel reproduced by Valerie Steele (1999: 6) two grown women admire a fashionable doll; there is not a child in sight. Behind the women is a romantic gothic-style building, clearly aristocratic in its park-like setting and the residence of one or both of the women. This plate was pirated in America by *Godey's Ladies Book*, but what is particularly curious is that there are children amongst the new figures, no doubt – as Steele indicates (1999: 4) – pirated from elsewhere, but the addition of the children firmly identifies the doll's purpose as 'toy'. In the original French print the doll only had an adult audience, suggesting that the Parisienne had currency amongst fashionable women as well as children. In another plate by Laure Noel from *Le Journal des Demoiselles et Petit Courier des Dames*, undated, but from c.1870–1875, the circle of similar fashions between the doll and the adult women is again represented, with the child in the middle wearing her own specific *mode enfantine* (see Figure 3.4). The doll's dress, when carefully scrutinised, combines the draped polonaise worn by the woman on the

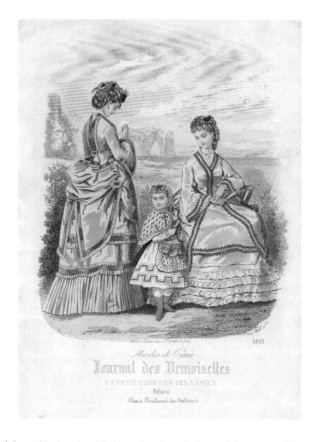

Figure 3.4 Laure Noel, undated fashion plate from *Le Journal des Demoiselles*, early-1870s.

left with the zigzag-edged lace that trims the dress of the woman on the right. In another plate from the same magazine, dated 1 March 1882,[3] the identity of the doll has shifted (see Figure 3.5). While her physicality is not so clearly defined as in Renoir's *Children's Afternoon*, her proportions are those of the stockier bébé, rather than the Parisienne. Her clothes are children's rather than adult fashions as her skirt is shorter than that worn by the doll drawn by Noel in the 1870s, and her loose and flowing hair is a girl's hairstyle rather than a woman's. The process of moving the acceptable ideal of the doll away from an image of high fashion to that of a baby to be mothered is under way. However here the doll is still placed in the public life of grand reception rooms, and the traffic of the generally accessible areas of the home, rather than the secluded domestic spaces as evidenced by the visible setting.

Emile-Louis Jumeau depicted his dolls as providing correct social instruction. They share in such rituals as *La Causette au Tuilleries*, according to an illustration

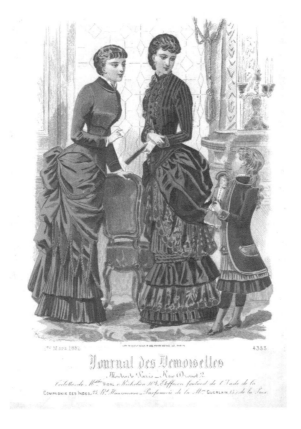

Figure 3.5 Artist unknown, fashion plate from *Le Journal des Demoiselles*, 1 March 1882.

in *Bébé Jumeau à L'Exposition*, 1889 (Anon 1889), seated on the child's lap whilst the fashionably dressed mothers talk. Not all the lives of Parisian dolls were so circumspect. A photograph by a Parisian photographer of c.1860 (see figure 3.2) shows a doll, whose high-waisted tartan crinoline clearly puts her in the accepted repertoire of Huret as now understood from surviving ensembles. She is being swung unceremoniously by her arm and sits astride another chair in a most undignified manner. The most fascinating aspect of the photographs is that the child has side-parted short hair, generally an indication of masculine gender. Girls had their hair cut during illness but generally kept their middle parting and this child is too sturdy for a *convalescente*. The dress itself, with ruching but no lace or flowers, falls within the canon for boyswear as evidenced by French fashion plates of the period. Fine German and French dolls, often dressed in naval or military uniforms, were regarded as appropriate boys' toys until the turn of the twentieth century, and there was a repertoire, especially from the 1860s, of finely dressed male Parisiens.

The casualness of the child's interaction with the fashionable doll may suggest a boy rather than a girl.

The adult usages of Parisiennes and French dolls are elusive. François Theimer has found a doll bearing a label, which indicated that it was wholesaled by the Jumeau firm, although the doll itself was a wax doll made in Britain. A handwritten notation in French on the doll's box also documents that it was a gift to a Gabrielle Detrenris on Coming of Age (twenty-first birthday; Theimer and Theriault 1994: 42–3). He states that in the 1840s customers for expensive French dolls were 'Haute Couture specialists, statesmen, or the nobility, eager to make a sumptuous presence by embodying French genius in high fashion' (Theimer and Theriault 1994: 32). 'It is certain that many of the "Parisian" or fashion dolls were never put into the hands of children' he further claims (Theimer and Theriault 1994: 83). French nineteenth-century custom included giving fashionable lady dolls to adult women, as wedding gifts and coming-of-age gifts. They were included as part of a bride's trousseau. A critique of the dolls at the 1867 Paris Exhibition says that they were given to women by men, potential lovers, who 'covered their intentions with the pretext of offering the present to the woman's young daughter'. (Theimer and Theriault 1994: 59) Another possible purpose for the dolls of questionable morality reported by Jules Delbruck was that the dolls were intended to instruct wealthy young girls on the verge of leaving the convent. All in all Delbruck thought that the dolls provided very unhealthy instruction to young girls. They were haughty as 'ladies in waiting' peering through their lorgnettes (Theimer and Theriault 1994: 59). The idea that the 'wrong' sort of doll brought an inappropriate sexual element into girls' lives pre-dates Barbie by at least a century. Often those who define or calibrate an 'appropriate' level of sexual content in a given doll are masculine, as with the department store buyers who rejected Barbie in 1959. Perhaps the issue being protected is male privilege as much as female purity?

The British journalist George Augustus Sala also regarded the French doll's luxury as excessive during this same exhibition year of 1867. He particularly deplored the multiplicity of objects made for the fictitious 'use' of the inanimate doll. Behind the criticism of the replication of useless objects is an inferred criticism of the rapaciousness of the seller and the gullibility of the consumer, who is exploited by the world of the fantasy life of the doll, created to encourage the purchasing of doll accessories. The mocking tone as the rational male looks at the irrational feminine world of the fashion doll is not only akin to the critiques directed against the Barbie doll, but also deeply misogynist. Not only is the *Marchande de Mode*, by implication, feminine, but the criticism of the fashion doll represents criticism of the female consumer of fashion. The translation of human objects and activities into doll scale is employed as a technique to further render women, their lifestyles and their patterns of consumption, ridiculous. Sala laments the simplicity of the past when longing for the unsophisticated 'rag-bran' (qtd

Theriault 1994: 7) stuffed dolls that once were produced, prior to the development of these artificial Parisiennes. Thus the idea that fashion wrongly overwrites the simple and innocuous nature of an essentialised femininity with a ridiculously artificial superstructure is long-standing. In the course of such arguments women are invariably imaged as incontinently susceptible to the superficial, delusory appeal of fashion. Conversely men, by their inferred ability to look through fashion's blandishments and recognise its specious nature, are imaged as intellectually superior.

> The doll's *Marchande de mode* discovered that dolly required a parasol, a pocket handkerchief, a reticule, a scent bottle and a huswife-case [sic] . . . Then they found out that she wanted a trunk, with a moveable tray, for her fine linen, a toilet table and looking glass, and brushes with ivory backs, a pack of cards to tell her fortune, a purse to hold her donations to the poor, a fan when she was warm, a railway rug symmetrically strapped up when she travelled, a prayer-book when she was pious and a birch rod when she was naughty. (qtd Theriault 1994: 7)

I have yet to see a birch rod in a Parisienne's trunk or trousseau. Sala's ironic addition of a birch rod to the list of objects produced by French dollmakers indicates that his ruminations upon the nature of women run to erotic fantasy and exaggerations.

A French report written at the time of the 1867 exhibition used the fashionable doll as a metaphor for defining the evils and moral shortcomings of modern life. The doll's lack of physical beauty was seen to guarantee a healthy and sane spirit in the agora. 'A dozen years ago [1855] Paris, and indeed the whole continent found content in the simple old fashioned dolls . . . with waxen . . . faces [and] with the blue shoes and the openwork socks . . . Dolly was a mere bifurcated bag of bran. Sometimes she had pink kid legs, but they were entirely innocent of calves' (source unknown; qtd Coleman et al. 1975: 104). Moreover she was an excellent example that encouraged economy and thrift in the young girls who made her clothes.

> In those unsophisticated times there prevailed a sensible custom, now all but extinct, of presenting children with undressed dolls. The happy possessor of the bag with the waxen extremities forthwith set up as a milliner and dressmaker on her own account . . . and many bitter tears were shed, I have no doubt, over bonnets and bodies that would never fit. But little girls learned to be neat and tidy and handy, which was something. (source unknown; qtd Coleman et al. 1975: 104)

The development of the luxury doll industry indicated for the above writer the corruption of modern society, and by implication the rottenness of the Second Empire. The doll precisely steps into the shoes of the *grande horizontale*.

I have always thought that the chief offender in bringing about that which I cannot but consider a decline of manners and a corruption of taste was a person who soon after the Crimean War, started a doll's wardrobe shop on the Rue de Choiseul. The shop was a very little one, and the stock in trade of a similarly diminutive nature. The whole display was extravagantly absurd, but irresistibly fascinating . . . This shop in the Rue de Choiseul was the parent of at least two hundred establishments of a similar nature which are now [1867] scattered all over Paris. (source unknown; qtd Coleman et al. 1975: 104)

As the Colemans point out, there were so many dolls' couturiers on the Rue de Choiseul in the 1850s and 1860s, including Au Bengali and Madame Lavallée-Peronne's A La Poupée de Nuremberg, that the company indicted as responsible for the explosion of useless luxury in the guise of dolls' fashions cannot be firmly identified.

Texts produced for women also regarded the French doll as allegorical of French style and fashion, but the attitudes towards the multiplication of novelties differed markedly. For the Parisian correspondent of the *Englishwoman's Domestic Magazine,* the fashion dolls were not to be deplored. They were 'interesting demoiselles' whose 'trousseaux are marvels of splendour and costliness'.

Dressing dolls is no mean employment in Paris; there are special couturiers for this branch of fashion and all the newest models are conscientiously copied for them. As for bonnets, they have choice of which one may judge by the fact that above four hundred models have been prepared. We are very far from the baby doll which its little girl mother was so happy to dress in a clean white frock and a blue sash. The modern doll is no baby; it is a lady of fashion, dressed up in a puff and a train, with Angot bonnet and Louis Quinze boots, who carries a glass in her eye, and a poodle dog under her arm in imitation of – well! Not of the elite of elegant women. ('Our Paris Letter', *English-woman's Domestic Magazine*, volume 20, January 1876, p. 79; qtd Johnston 1986: 66)

Like G.A. Sala, this anonymous writer also places the modern French doll with her vast trousseau of up-to-date novelties against the artless and plain dolls of the past. In this instance the superseded, plain dolls are explicitly identified as having a domestic identity. As 'baby' dolls, unlike the 'modern doll', the dolls of the past were *unfashionable* in their 'clean white frocks'. The cleanliness was also indicative of household diligence. The simplicity of their garb, 'clean white frock and a blue sash', also places fashion in opposition to the virtues of homemaking.

This tension between 'fashion' and the modesty of acceptable female behaviour is further highlighted in later sections of this report on the latest doll novelties. After having luxuriated in details of the variety and elaboration of doll fashions in Paris, the writer declares 'if the doll of the period is no baby, the little girl of the period is no child'. For any British Victorian reader, the concept of the 'doll of the period' would have immediately brought to mind 'the Girl of the Period'. This was a catchphrase from a journalistic controversy instituted by Mrs Lynn Linton who in a famed essay in the *Saturday Review* in 1868 deplored the fact that decent, young English girls slavishly followed fashions set by Parisian courtesans. She further asserted that the love of dress leads to fastness, slangish talk and indifference to duty (Hughes 2000: 113–14; Linton 2003). This reference to the 'Girl of the Period' immediately evokes Paris and high fashion, as well as the pitfalls that were supposed to derive for modest womanhood from overly assiduous devotion to those dual false gods of Paris and fashion. If a girl intended to use fashion to gain a husband, then she may fail, as men flirt with these new bold and slangy women, but never marry them. Claire Hughes indicates that a 'strain of fairly crude xenophobia' runs through Linton's essay (2000: 114), but the controversy, as much as it sought to limit the influence of new and vulgar fashion on impressionable young girls, also acted as an effectively comprehensive textbook to any aspiring stylist as to how to be modern. The issue was debated internationally through cartoons, songs, sketches and parodies. Various consumer goods including parasols and cigars were advertised as being 'of the period' (2000: 113–14).

The reference to the French fashion doll being 'the doll of the period' not only places her within this vocabulary of fashionable marketing of the 1860s and early-1870s, but also immediately conjures up this conjunction of newly rebellious womanhood, the refusal of the angel of the house, high fashion and the visible prostitution of the Second Empire. Part of the immorality of these forward young women was their use of false beauty aids, cosmetics, hairpieces, hair dyes, and artificial fashions. Indeed young women with fashionable aspirations were making not only cocottes but also dolls of themselves, insofar as formerly modest, natural 'girls' were now constructed as the sum of simulcra and prostheses. Placed at the end of a long passage glorifying the Parisian doll as a replica of high fashion, and the divine madness and expense of all that could be bought for her, the final critique of both the dolls, and those who bought them, seems to be an opportunistic and belated turn of mind towards moralising for the *Englishwoman's Domestic Magazine*. If the writer fears that hardly one genuine child still existed in France, as evidenced by the lack of genuine, homely dolls, the Parisienne doll becomes a conduit by which unease and uncertainties about movements and advances in female position could be publicly debated. These metaphors are all deeply familiar to anyone who has traced discussion of the Barbie doll. It is not only in her slim adult proportions and her fashionable wardrobe that the Parisienne is a Barbie avatar.

Pretty, Magnificent, Wonderful: the French Bébé and Female Representation

Understand me well, I shall never learn anything. I am pretty, magnificent, wonderful, but unfortunately I am not intelligent.

Thus did the iconic late-nineteenth-century doll of choice, Bébé Jumeau, introduce herself in a 'letter' to her potential owner, which was included as advertising material in her box (qtd Melger 1997: 41). No date is given for this document, quoted by a doll historian, but other Jumeau advertising booklets date generally from the 1880–1890 period. Bébé Jumeau further outlined her singular and perfect nature as woman and, by inference, catalogued the common faults of her less-gifted living sisters.

I have promised myself many happy days in your company. I will be obedient and sociable and above all so undemanding of you that you shall quickly find me dear to you, because I do not want to be your loving, unbreakable doll, but also a friend who knows how to console you when your heart is heavy from difficulties. In addition to obedience, I have many other qualities which set me apart from other babies. Firstly I am discreet and most of all deaf and dumb since my birth, so that you can count on me never repeating your words to anyone or gossiping about anything you may have done. My large blue eyes which shine so beautifully, will never betray my emotions. [punctuation sic] (qtd Melger 1997: 40)

Cherished throughout the twentieth century and into the twenty-first by doll collectors, who will pay tens of thousands of US dollars at auction for superlative examples, and acquired internationally by certain museums as adjuncts to collections of historic dress or social history records of 'childhood', the late-nineteenth-century French bébé is both entirely expressive of the strange, profound and anxious scrutiny of women during the Third Republic and virtually invisible in academic deconstructions and analyses of this representation of women. This chapter surveys the intersection of the bébé as cultural artefact with current scholarship on women, sexuality, visibility and fashion.

The bébé doll is not literally the baby that the direct translation of her name implies. Baby dolls, ubiquitous in the twentieth century, were relatively infrequent

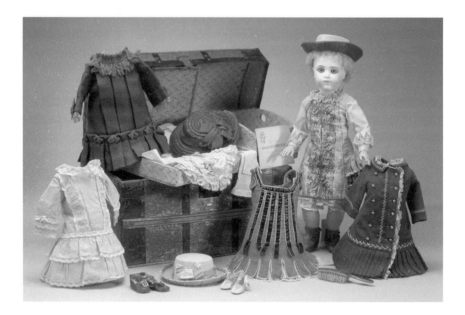

Figure 4.1 Rare early wooden-bodied Bébé Bru c.1880, with original trousseau by Appolyne Bru, formerly in collection of Maurine Popp, image by courtesy of Skinners Auctions, USA.

in the nineteenth. The term bébé evolved in the late-1870s to indicate that she had a younger persona than the fashionable Parisienne. Whilst some bébés are found dressed in infants' long clothes, the majority represent girls between the ages of two and twelve years old. Leon Casimir Bru's bébés appear to be a little older: up to fifteen years old. Occasionally bébés are found dressed in adult female clothes, particularly those wearing ethnic and folkloric clothing. Bébés dressed by home dressmakers or beyond Parisian ateliers also often wear adult styles.

The bébé takes the story of the French Haute Couture doll from its heyday in the 1870s up to its disappearance at the turn of the century. Although forgotten by fashion historians, the bébé assisted in the diffusion of French fashion in the late-nineteenth century and generated popular perceptions of fashion. She documents foundational elements of the commodification and mass marketing of high fashion images, and the formalisation of new channels of information about style in late-nineteenth-century France. Alongside other media, dolls facilitated this modernisation of communication around fashion.

The bébé extended the marketing and industrial practices established for the Parisienne even further, but ultimately moved beyond direct connection with fashion. Finally the whole bébé phenomenon evaporated its Haute Couture cross-references under pressure from commercialisation and mass production. At this point, the dollmaking aesthetic could not sustain the level of quality in construction and detailing that would justify the products being regarded as an extension of the French high fashion industry.

Fashion Marketing and Modernity: the Jumeau Firm as Avatar and Case Study

The bébé illuminates the rapid consolidation of fashion in Anglo-European culture into industrial practice, the commodification and mass marketing of an image of high fashion luxury and the development of a quasi-industrial system for selling high fashion. Thus the bébé is an essential component of the history of the modern fashion doll boom. If Huret pre-dated Worth in the technique of spinning out, and then capitalising upon reputation in the elusive field of fashion to create a concrete resource that could be marketed for profit, then the Jumeau company, in particular, indicates the future, vast cross marketing of style and leisure throughout the twentieth century. For many decades French luxury industries have been at the summit of the scale of purchasing and desire, not only within couture, but also the more affordable, broader marketplace of mass-produced licensed products such as perfumes and scarves. The Jumeau firm perfected the international marketing of 'style' a century before it became commonplace in the fashion industry.

If we are contemplating 'Barbie' as a phenomenon, the French bébé as a genre proves a particularly rich prehistory to the issues of branding and marketing both dolls and an image of 'fashion'. The bébé suggests that these phenomena were articulated about a century earlier than Superstar Barbie of 1977. The flexibility and universality of the Jumeau firm makes it a prequel to the Mattel firm, which both academic and collector literature treats as standing alone. Bébé Jumeau also endows the French expertise in marketing style and luxury with a history. Behind the modern conglomerates of style retailing, behind Vuitton, Saint Laurent and the licensed product, stands the Jumeau firm; a high level of industrial production was achieved, turning out a staggering three million dolls a year by the 1890s. Many of these dolls were dressed in 'couturier' fashions designed by Ernestine Jumeau and executed by her more than 200 atelier-based hands and outworkers, without lowering the reputation of the Jumeau name as a byword of style and elegance until the late-1890s.

The firm's flexible, versatile stratagems and the interlocking elements of its activities make it an important early case study for historians of fashion and style marketing. No dollmaking contemporaries in Paris matched the modernity and range of either confident socio-cultural self-placement or techniques of promotion and production, and few couturiers of the 1880s for adult fashion fully shared the industrial confidence and scale of the Jumeau firm. If Paul Poiret is renowned in conventional fashion history for making the name of his studio newsworthy

(Mackrell 1990: 12, 81) and proclaiming his product as an essential expression of the ethos of his era, two decades earlier Jumeau certainly intruded into the public life of his contemporaries with the marketing of a product renowned for its quint-essential 'style'. Remarkably, despite the vast size of his production, Emile-Louis Jumeau claimed for his products and his atelier the same singular, exclusive, avant-garde status of a couture house. If, like Nancy Troy, one takes Worth and Poiret as case studies for the uneasy relations between original and copy, creativity and productivity in Haute Couture (2003: 4–16, 20–25), the Jumeau company should also be considered a site where new concepts of fashion marketing were tested in the marketplace. Emile-Louis Jumeau stood head and shoulders above his rivals in the toy and fashion industries by the universal scale of his ambitious programme to insinuate his products into the supposedly transparent 'naturalness' of the rule of taste. The activities of the Jumeau company overshadowed the whole genre of the bébé and set the pace for its competitors, who remained essentially reactive. Indeed beyond the Jumeau dolls the others – no matter how beautiful in aesthetic terms or how much collectors will pay for them – are mere accessories as cultural signs to the fact of the Jumeau bébé. She is the paradigm of the remarkable art genre of luxurious French child dolls.

In the nineteenth century, Bébé Jumeau lived as a character through sheet music, children's stories, pamphlets, engravings, lithographs and cunningly planted copy in adult print media.[1] The most notable of the promotional materials around Bébé Jumeau was the 1889 board game in which she escaped the Germans and climbed the Eiffel Tower. Her universal, inescapable presence, and the range of means by which she was integrated into the child's psyche, prefigures twentieth-century 'character merchandising'. Bébé Jumeau was not perhaps as fixed and final as the present-day cartoon characters in product merchandising. These modern characters' metamorphosis from the abstraction of story or illustration to a concrete three-dimensional product – such as a Barbie-sized doll – follows a very direct trajectory. The known, fixed appearance and narrative around the character is essential to this process and ensures the success of the migration from medium to medium. Disney's Belle, to take an example at random, never changes her appearance, whereas Bébé Jumeau, even when dressed by the company, has a multiplicity of looks. By the mid-1880s, the firm proudly boasted of originating more than three hundred original couture models a year (Cusset 1957: 58). Exact replicas of Jumeau dresses on two dolls from different provenances are seldom found, unless they are the standard garments that the non-couture dolls wore on leaving the factory; even these 'standard' dolls sometimes survive in their original boxes with extra, individualised accessories from the company, such as quality gloves or hats. Only the 'twin' dolls, which the company produced as a novelty, provide exact copies of a model, sometimes the same dress trimmed with ribbons in two different colours. Conversely, with Disney's Belle our recognition that her yellow dress is not Cinderella's blue dress or Sleeping Beauty's pink dress, or equally our recognition that her chestnut brown hair is not Ariel's red hair establishes her identity in the eye of the beholder and authenticates the 'merchandise' which her fans may wish to buy. The Worth company had to face up to the danger of self-repetition and seemed to have managed it with more stress than did the Jumeau company. Worth's atelier had to maintain a complex indexing system to ensure that different women did not turn up to the same function in the same garment (Troy 2003: 22). With the 'Disney Princesses' repetition is not a pitfall but a guarantee of each characters' reality against her imitators, even though the 'Princesses' therefore exist in most un-regal profusion.

Bébé Jumeau is never so fixed in her representation as to be identifiable by colour and pen stroke. Both Carl Fox and Stuart Holbrook testify to the multiplicity of identities and faces that Bébé Jumeau may have within the catchment of her 'beauty'. According to Holbrook, when seen en masse, each Bébé Jumeau's individual beauty proves that she is an artistic rather than a production item (1990: 32–3). For Fox, Bébé Jumeau's beauty shines through the homeliest disguises. She has many expressions, but the fact of her femininity does not change.

> Legends die hard, but the legendary beauty of Jumeau's numerous lady dolls and bébés cannot be questioned. Their appeal is universal. Wherever Jumeau dolls were exhibited – Paris, London, Vienna, Philadelphia, New Orleans, Melbourne – gold medals and diplomas were showered on these loveliest of bisque dolls. Other dolls may have more character, look more or less realistic, look like your baby, a child next door; for me the physical beauty of Jumeau's dolls has not been surpassed. (Fox 1972: 27)

> Even in the most nondescript clothing bisque Jumeau bébés have a seductive charm a consistent beauty. In reviewing the long history of dolls, I find the Jumeaus most agreeable, their standard of beauty, to my western eyes most easy to accept. They are like early Renoir paintings of young ladies, pretty but not saccharine. (1972: 213)

He even likens one individual Bébé Jumeau to the 'ravishing arrogance' of the young Simone Signoret (1972: 115), thus moving the relatively arcane Bébé Jumeau rightfully into the spotlight of the modern star system. He links this Jumeau doll to a particular woman, renowned not only as attractive, but also as intellectually and politically responsible. Signoret was understood to be proudly Other to the 'mindless' stars of Hollywood and, as a political thinker, she was also beyond the McCarthy witch hunts. Fox's comparison is one of the few modern – or politically orientated – analogies made around French bébés in doll literature.

The Jumeau doll represents the laissez-faire infancy of merchandising and branding; her identity is loosely interpreted and appearance is not fixed as an essential tool of the marketing process. Yet Emile-Louis Jumeau seems to have grasped the basic principles of product placement and the integrated marketing of entertainment and style a century before it became commonplace. Such marketing strategies are read as a sign of North American culture overwriting all others. Perhaps one could regard 'Eurodisney' as a high point of American cultural imperialism – indeed one could say that the recent Disney epics had strong meanings, 'sources, context, target', specially directed to Europe (Byrne and McQuillan 1999: 21): the *Little Mermaid*, 1989, with its hard lessons about obligation and debt, and the dangers of longing for an alien paradise, for Eastern Europe (1999: 22–36); and *Beauty and the Beast*, 1991, for Western Europe, protective of its cultural maturity in comparison to the USA. Ironically, in view of the intellectual misgivings around the Disney corporation's homogenising impetus and its imperial expansion into the imagination, the Jumeau firm provides a European precedent and origin for character merchandising and integrated marketing of 'play' as 'product'.

The consistent modernity of the Bébé Jumeau phenomenon never fails. The English translation of the French play *La Poupée* – a popular theatrical piece – at its 1890s premiere American production became an early example of cross marketing and product placement. *La Poupée* concerned a doll to whom a Catholic prelate needed to be 'married' in order for him to gain an inheritance but concurrently maintain his vows of celibacy. French dollmakers' imitation of female life resonated with the essentialised passivity and artificiality of female nature in cultural constructs to lend the plot satiric credibility. Actress Anna Held, who played the doll, was supposed to resemble a Bébé Jumeau to such a degree that the cunning publicity machine around the actress claimed that it would be no surprise if she were tattooed with the Jumeau brandname (Golden 2000: 36). Held prefigured a number of late-twentieth-century women, from collectors to performance artists, who, a century later, have aspired to 'be' Barbie, to look like, to live as Barbie, either permanently or temporarily, for a performance or an event (Rogers 1999: 21). The Sindy doll is also celebrated by English performers and friends (Page 1988: 114). In a number of countries Mattel employs young women, often fashion models or actresses between assignments, as 'living Barbies', who host tea parties and promotions in department stores and shopping malls, dressed in adult-scale reproductions of Barbie clothes (Lalli 1986: 138–40). The modernity of the Jumeau experience in terms of branding and marketing is once again clear.

Jumeau was both an exemplary bourgeois capitalist – hard-working, self-motivated, entrepreneurial – and a social transgressor because he refused to keep to his place in class/social hierarchies. Jumeau desired – and achieved – upper-class status for himself and his family. Conversely, Worth always remained an outsider, potentially tainted by the dangerous knowledge of his association with his clients' bodies (Troy 2003: 28). For Jumeau, unlike Worth, this disturbing, intrusive knowledge of female bodies was mediated through the third party of the doll. Jumeau accrued and maintained a fortune, moving to the photographic trade in the late-nineteenth century, when dollmaking was undermined by German mass production. Before the rapid decline of the French doll trade in the 1890s, he received the Légion d'Honneur in 1886 for his achievements as businessman and patriot, based solely upon manufacturing and exporting luxury porcelain dolls. Police reports on his character and morals castigate him not for any sexual misdemeanours, but for living ostentatiously above his station (Theimer and Theriault 1994: 121–6). From surviving evidence, Jumeau appears to have been text-and-discourse-driven in a manner that rendered him a paradigm of French intellectual Enlightenment obsessions of the Third Republic – scientific, social, sexual, nationalist. These discourses are possibly rendered more unambiguous because the speaker had come from beyond the boundaries of couth intellectual society, and his creation could be perceived to be marginal, ludicrous, out of proportion to his ambition. Jumeau and his dolls are parodic expressions of the central myth of the Enlightenment male creator.

Jumeau represented himself throughout advertising brochures and press interviews/accounts in a number of guises. He claimed to have originally trained as an architect but – martyr-like – accepted the humiliating return (further down the class hierarchy towards the artisanal) to the family dollmaking business (Cusset 1957: 61, 65) when his elder brother (and natural heir to the company) died in 1872. Familial duty called and Jumeau gained virtu in heeding – against his own desires and ambitions – the rules of a more eternal order: the family. As the French state from the eighteenth century onwards was itself often represented through the metaphor of the French household/family under the wise counsel of the leader-father (Merrick 1990: 68–84), here is probably yet another enactment of Jumeau's highly obvious professions of loyalty to the French nation. However, recent French research suggests that Jumeau never had professional architectural training and was working in the doll company from before the years of his majority (Theimer and Theriault 1994: 71). Like Coco Chanel a generation later, Jumeau was perhaps circulating more presentable origin myths about himself to facilitate a smoother integration amongst his cultural (if not class) peers in French society.

In some accounts he presents himself as the ultimate scientific discoverer, a man of insight and high standards like Pasteur or Charcot, frustrated by his lower-class workers' bumbling attempts to render his enlightened, informed vision into reality.

> Many and many a time he threw aside imperfect babies which he deemed unworthy of being offered to pretty little misses such as you; many and many a time he was seen to tear his hair in fits of passion and indignation at being so sorely misunderstood by work-people who delivered uncouth, caricature-like babies. Years of unceasing efforts have been necessary to make us what we are, the king of babies. (Anon c.1880: np)

Jumeau rendered himself a more complete citizen by peforming positivist discourses and claiming that his personal economic advancement and stratagems were a public/patriotic service underpinning his noble and public-minded spirit.

> Playthings are of no less interest from the industrial point of view than they are from the scientific point of view, as will be seen from this article. Before the visit that we had the opportunity to make to the famous doll factory at Montreuil, near Paris, we failed to suspect the magnitude that can be achieved by this very special type of industry. The director and founder of this factory, Mr Jumeau, whose name is universally known, did us the honour of showing us his establishment with most gracious courtesy . . . we are going to impart to our readers our surprise in fact our amazement – at seeing such well organised production . . . it is the largest doll factory in the entire world . . . (Gaston Tissandier 'The Parisian Industries: A Doll Factory', in *La Nature* 1888; qtd Whitton 1980: 19)

Jumeau the industrialist is not merely 'universally known', but also comports himself as if he were a gentleman and showed visitors around the doll factory 'with most gracious courtesy'. As 'the largest doll factory in the entire world', Jumeau's manufacturing plant played a role in upholding and symbolising French prestige and singularity.

> M. Jumeau 'artisan de sa fortune' does not only contribute to the well being of those numerous families who work in his industry, he has given to his country a fertile source of revenue, which grows daily in importance . . . The magnificent establishment which he founded in Montreuil is a model city, where over three hundred workers are hardly enough to serve the market, where the order, the work, the system, and the activity present a spectacle that is one of the most pleasurable that can be contemplated. (*La France*, 15 December 1884; qtd Theimer and Theriault 1994: 113)

The system and the act of industrialisation are praised for their own sakes, causing an aesthetic frisson. Moreover Jumeau's individual act of capitalist endeavour in building up the factory is seen to reflect credibly on a broader community.

Jumeau's most important public service was possibly the regulation of womanhood. Through his activities as dollmaker, this correction of female aberrances could take place at all levels of society. In the middle and upper classes the allure of the Jumeau doll, and therefore the potential reward of a gift of a doll, encouraged young girls to improve their behaviour. Conversely young girls' negotiations to get a doll bought for them were also exercises in appropriate feminine behaviour – wheedling and flirtation. Advertising booklets put out by Jumeau frequently include this scene of the female child demanding a doll and negotiating and striking bargains:

– Mamma Mamma, I should like a Jumeau baby.
– When you are good I shall buy you one.
– Why not at once, mother dear? rejoined the child coaxingly.
– Because such a handsome baby is given only to studious and obedient children and, as you are far from combining these two qualities I refuse.
– Oh Mamma I promise to amend my faults if you give it me [sic].
– Amend yourself first, and I shall afford that pleasure afterwards.
Well I can assure you that, from their anxiety to secure our possession many little girls became so good that their parents were quite surprised and soon made them a present of one of us. (Anon c.1880: np)

Marie . . . turned towards her mother.
– Oh Mamma, when will I have a Bébé Jumeau?
– Tomorrow if you promise to follow the teaching and example that it gives you.
– Yes Mamma, I swear to you I will. (Anon c.1889: np)

With the working classes Jumeau intervened more directly. Readers are informed that he put himself at considerable expense to pay his women workers above average pay because he realised that poor wages encouraged women to go on the streets.

Women's work, as is well known, is very badly paid. Monsieur Jumeau has reacted against this bad habit the cause of so many fallen women, alas! He has given himself the unrewarding task of employing as many women as possible in his factory. He pays them a good salary. Owing to the work being well paid, one cannot accuse Monsieur Jumeau of having thought to find cheap labour by employing mostly women. (Cusset 1957: 12)

Ironically, despite the inherently patriarchal imagery, the success of the Jumeau company was partly due to the exertions and skills of Ernestine Jumeau, Jumeau's wife, who – even as the company disseminated images of wheedling, astute daughters and the fortuitous diversion of potential prostitutes – was responsible for running half the company in the city showroom in Paris. She controlled the workrooms for dressing, packing and shipping the dolls and she supervised around fifty hands in the atelier and over two hundred outworkers (Whitton 1980: 8). The dresses and final appearance of the dolls, which contributed significantly to the appeal of the Jumeau doll, were Ernestine's responsibility. She worked after the birth of her three daughters, leaving the house to be run by servants, whom she briefed each morning (Theimer and Theriault 1994: 6), and leaving the daughters – apparently, to the delight of visitors, frequently dressed in the same dresses as their father's dolls (Theimer and Theriault 1994: 111) – to be educated by governesses. Perhaps the artisanal and craft origins of the Jumeau firm permitted a pre-industrial-revolution division of gender roles within the family, where female labour, in partnership with male labour in the household, made a positive and necessary contribution to the overall economic viability of the family unit.

Jumeau himself sees the philosophical link between the family and the French state. He likens the world of fashion that his wife creates to an old vision of France, a kingdom, where Madame Jumeau held morning *levée* just like the *Roi Soleil* himself. She also wields the power of the newly emerged couturiers such as Worth.

> We have been transported into a kingdom where clothes wave the sceptre, and this state is reigned over by Madame Jumeau, who brings to her task her impeccable taste, her perfect elegance and her love of beauty. Every morning she holds her court and receives her workers, who bring to her their latest models in hats and clothes. It is a task to which the workers, with fairy fingers, put all their energy. Many children of millionaires do not have more beautiful clothes than the Bébé Jumeau. The colours are artistically blended, the silks and satin of the clothes and the laces and ribbons are skilfully blended to form an artistic whole. (Cusset 1957: 56–7)

Cusset further claims that the Jumeau company was comparable to a major fashion house in the scale of its production. It was a leading customer of Lyons silk merchants and bought directly from lace and textile manufacturers (1957: 57). Labelling on the dolls' boxes indicates that there was a lower-priced line of dolls fashionably dressed in second-hand silk. How strange that the doll may have been dressed in silks cast off from either a society lady or a courtesan.

The Jumeau company was seen as comparable to an adult couture house in keeping up with the latest modes to produce garments in the best of taste.

> I have seen dresses which have taken eight days to complete. The most wonderful ball dress would not take longer to make. I have gone into ecstasies over exquisite suits and hats of the greatest taste and elegance.
>
> The shops of the Rue Pastourelle really show the latest novelties. The materials come direct from the makers, and I can assure you that the House of Jumeau is considered an important client. Then there are the feathers for the hats, the shoe laces and the shoes, the silk stockings, the petticoats, the gloves and in fact the whole trousseau, as complicated and refined as that of the most elegant coquette. (Cusset 1957: 57)

Theimer, perhaps quoting Jumeau family recollections, claims for Ernestine Jumeau a high reputation amongst her Parisian contemporaries as an expert couturière. 'Her grace and elegance were much admired by journalists' (Theimer and Theriault 1994: 168), whilst her mind was 'open and resolutely modern' (Theimer and Theriault 1994: 70). The idea that Jumeau did not follow, but led, current fashion, or even acted as a predictor and trendsetter, appeared in a number of sources. The dolls were 'dressed in the latest fashion, and even that of tomorrow, for here one does not follow the fashion, one creates it' (Cusset 1957: 56). The

American report on the 1889 exhibition claimed of Jumeau's dolls that 'perhaps they have even set the fashion sometimes; if so, the best dressmakers of the day need not be ashamed' (Coleman et al. 1970: 335).

The Bébé Trade in Paris

The Bru company was a smaller, more artisanal studio. It stayed loyal to the Parisienne's kid body, often made under contract by Jumeau (Theimer 1991: 67; Theimer and Theriault 1994: 200). In advertising, Bru always emphasised the artistic nature of his product and his small-scale enterprise. He consciously invoked issues of taste and style, which left nothing to desire – '*le cachet, l'élégance et la coquetterie ne laissent rien à désirer*' as described in his 1872 catalogue (Theimer 1991: 42) – to distinguish his firm from the industrially scaled Jumeau company. The Bru firm achieved some of its highest awards after the founder had sold the company to Henri Chevrot in 1883. Chevrot's advertising spoke of the Bru doll as being the best product on offer amongst all the Parisian bébés. Once again, the competitor was not named, but the Bru dolls were indicated as being superior in their construction as objects ('*le plus gracieux . . . de tous les Bébés Parisiens*' Theimer 1991: 107) in that they were the 'most solid and best jointed' of Parisian dolls, and also the most graceful, and therefore they were superior in style as well. Chevrot promoted his dolls through photographic trade cards that show male and female couples dressed by his studio in various guises: Spaniards, eighteenth-century rural workers and a high society bridal couple. All these dolls were in the bébé format, but were dressed sumptuously as adults. On the printed reverse of these cards Chevrot claimed that the Bébé Bru was a 'truly artistic toy, the most perfect of all bébés', adopted unequivocally by people of taste.

If one can try to predict or identify a house style amongst bébés' wardrobes, the Jumeau company had, amongst the general diversity of their so-called 'couture' ensembles (collectors' terminology for the finely detailed and finished clothing of Jumeau's best grade of dolls) a number of characteristic looks. These include dresses in silk brocades, usually pastel shades, such as pinks, blues, aquamarine, creams (see Figure 4.2). Another series of dresses follows the 1880s interest in contrasting colours, maroons and creams being a recurring combination. The brown tonalities that were favoured in 1880s adultwear were also frequently seen in Jumeau dolls. A favoured format associated with the company by collectors, and now often published in modern pattern drafts as a 'Jumeau' dress, was a sleeveless dress, with a matching long-sleeved jacket to be worn over the sleeveless dress.

When put alongside known Jumeau dresses, there is a tendency for many Bru dresses to be cut from darker, more intense shades of fabrics, such as royal blues, ruby reds, deep wine reds. Whilst one should use the comparison with some

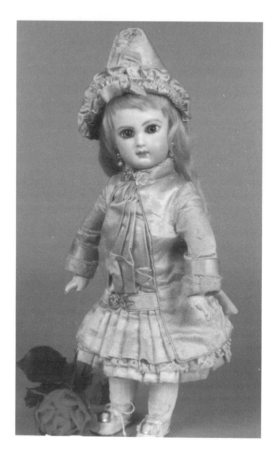

Figure 4.2 Bébé Jumeau in original outfit by Ernestine Jumeau mid-1880s, image by courtesy of McMasters Harris Auctions, USA.

caution, Bru dressing takes the same dramatic approach to fashion as did Worth, particularly the use of brocades and woven silks in eye-catching patterns, bold abstract designs or strong contrasts of tones. Conversely, the Jumeau dresses often feature brocades and silks in more subtle self-tones, damask-like patterns or floral sprigs in the monochrome weave. Bru dolls in original condition often wear one-piece princess-line dresses, very tightly cut and closely fitted to the doll, again suggesting that in the 1880s the Bru firm presented each doll as an individual studio production. The detailing in the Bru dressing, of piping, of binding, of layers of ruffles, of trimmings, even exceeds that of Jumeau dolls (see Figure 4.3). Original Bru dresses show faultless technical construction. The first designer of Bru costuming, Madame Appolyne Bru, was the daughter of a master tailor and herself had worked as a professional seamstress, sewing for an undertaker in Paris. Advertising for the Bru company under the director Chevrot stated that the Bébé

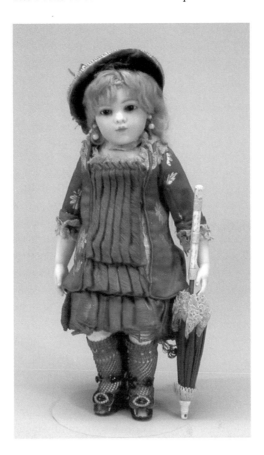

Figure 4.3 Bébé Bru in original outfit by Appolyne Bru early- to mid-1880s, formerly in collection of Maurine Popp, image by courtesy of Skinners Auctions, USA.

Brus were 'always elegantly dressed and in the latest fashion', and that because of the quality of their fashions and their *costumes de fantasie trés variés* Bébé Brus were chosen by *tous les personnes de gout*, all the people of taste.

Perhaps only the Steiner firm, with its astonishing range of inventions and mechanised figures, could match the Jumeau label for the detail and vividness of the picture that it paints of the society in which it is created, and the paradoxes of the female image that it created. The inventions of Jules Nicholas Steiner, whose doll production originated from a clockmaking skill base (McGonagle 1988: 8–11), could not more perfectly reflect postmodernist fascination with images and theories of gender, unless they had been devised as elements of a present-day postgraduate art major or an exhibition project. Steiner launched the widest range of different face sculptings amongst Paris-based dollmakers, including dolls with double rows of teeth resembling a closed Venus Flytrap, precursors to the *vagina dentatis*, which obsessed so many avant-garde artists of the early twentieth century. Steiner's Bébé Gigoteur, made from the 1850s to the 1900s, particularly presents women as *unheimlich*, disturbed and unnatural. Supposedly an infant doll, but often dressed as a child or a lady, one winds her key and she throws a fit, kicking her legs and feet, flailing her arms, twisting her head and crying. Steiner also produced dolls with segmented bodies, alternating cloth and porcelain, including perfectly moulded porcelain pelvises that inspire a fetishistic contemplation of the graceful, detailed modelling of the ceramic body parts. A 'waltzing lady' devised by Steiner also throws her arms up, cries and squeaks. These waltzing ladies can be dated from between the 1860s and 1890s, according to the shape of the cardboard skirt under which her clockwork mechanism is hidden. The contours of these cardboard skirts follow fashionable outline from the crinoline to the bustle.

The Steiner company did not achieve the level of public marketplace saturation that Jumeau did. It was a wholesale house and its products were known to the public in the guise of their retailers, rather than the manufacturer. The Parisian toy shop Au Nain Bleu was a major customer of the Steiner company (McGonagle 1988: 16). Many Steiner dolls and their garments have been found with Au Nain Bleu labels. Steiner mechanical dolls dating from c.1867 have been recorded with labels consigning them to other French doll companies including Jumeau and Terrène (McGonagle 1988: 12). Like the Bru company, the Steiner firm passed through a number of hands, and the high standards were eroded during the directorship of individuals with less inventive or insightful approaches to dollmaking, dressing and design. The fortunes and image of the Jumeau company drew strength from the consistent leadership over six decades by family members: Jumeau *père et fils*, and Madame Ernestine Jumeau.

The major Paris-based firms producing large quantities of bébés were Jumeau, Bru, Steiner and Gaultier. Gaultier bébés –like Gaultier's Parisiennes – bore the firm's initials but were never marketed as Bébé Gaultier, being sold on to other doll marketers. Gesland was one of the few buyers of Gaultier heads who placed his own trademark on the body. Collectors have elevated some dolls from smaller studios, such as the Thullier doll and the 'H-doll', to the forefront of bébé production and will pay excessive sums for these dolls on account of the small number of surviving dolls. H-dolls are now generally assigned to the maker Halopeau (Seeley 1992: 35), who took over the Barrois firm. The difference between bébés in style and quality is actually relatively small between the premium and ordinary examples, which command far lower prices. Unlike twentieth-century couture garments, which were admired and highly desired when made and have remained so, the high status assigned by later collectors to certain dolls does not necessarily follow the opinion of consumers at the time of manufacture. The star companies in early literature were the high-profile ones. The size and industrial efficiency of the Jumeau concern commended it to contemporary journalists. Emile-Louis Jumeau assiduously courted the press with great effectiveness. Again his instinctive grasp of changing social and cultural paradigms is apparent. For a cultural historian, André Jean Thullier's oeuvre is far blander and less informative than Emile-Louis Jumeau's. Rather than specific cultural merit or message, the high prices of Thullier's dolls speak of collectors' obsession with status denoted by price and the fetishistic frenzy of modern 'collectables'.

Most companies who produced bébés operated on a smaller scale than Jumeau's industrial orientation. These smaller companies do not appear to have sought the limelight as artistic and creative entities, nor to have encouraged a personality cult around their product. A French writer, Pierre du Maroussem, stated in 1894 that the Parisian doll trade consisted of three levels. There was small-scale studio production, assemblers of parts sourced from different manufacturers and finally industrial manufacturers. Maroussem claimed that only three companies, Jumeau, Steiner and Danel – this last company was founded by disaffected Jumeau employees – could be ranked as industrial concerns (qtd McGonagle 1988: 16). Other companies making bébés in smaller quantities include Halopeau, André Jean Thullier, Gesland, Schmitt et Fils, May Frères (whose Bébé Mascotte was named after a favourite *opera bouffe*, La Mascotte), Henri Alexandre, Henri Delcroix, Henri Danel, Alexandre Mothereau, Joseph Joanny, Rabery and Delphieu, and Petit and Dumontier.

If a line were to be drawn between the play doll and the fashionable bébé, it could be drawn at Rabery and Delphieu. Their dolls are not quite as good quality as other bébés in the substance of their bisque. The porcelain clay is grainier in texture, with dark sooty fragments amongst the white slip, but they are skilfully painted. Rabery dolls' big eyes and Cupid's bow lips follow the characteristic 'look' of elite French dolls. Rabery was a two-generational family company that made inexpensive dolls in mid-nineteenth-century Paris, often budget-priced lady dolls on cloth bodies, which steadily raised production values to emerge thirty years later and receive a gold medal for luxury bébés at the 1888 Antwerp Exhibition (Theimer 1993a: 153). They are frequently found in lavish dressing and, like Steiner dolls, Rabery and Delphieu's open-mouthed dolls are often as finely costumed as their closed-mouthed dolls. One that was illustrated by British dealer Kay Desmonde in her small album of antique dolls (Desmonde 1972: 40), wore a lemon-coloured brocade dress and hat in the 1890s romantic revival style of vaguely 1830s style fashions associated with popular artists such as Lucien Leandre. Another open-mouthed Rabery doll wears a well-tailored princess-line dress in brown velvet with royal purple satin facings from c.1880. Fully interfaced with hand-finished raw edges this dress is the standard expected of the best quality dolls' garments from 1880s Paris and exactly matches the techniques used in adult dressmaking. The Rabery doll was proud of her origins and her pedigree as a representative of the city of fashion; she was marketed under the trade name Bébé de Paris. This name appeared on her box rather than on any trademarks placed on the dolls.

Danel's Paris-Bébé sprang from industrial espionage. Danel was a disaffected employee of Jumeau, who stole some moulds for porcelain heads, and together with Monsieur Guepratte, Jumeau's shoemaker and eyemaker, produced a look-alike doll from the Jumeau moulds, with a patented spring-jointed body. The operation was closed down in 1892 after a protracted court battle in which Emile-Louis Jumeau managed to prove authorship of his dolls and the derivative nature of the Paris-Bébé (Theimer and Theriault 1994: 145–54). Jumeau took over the trademark and manufactured dolls under the name Paris-Bébé which indicated that his doll was the soul of the city of fashion itself. Danel had chosen the Eiffel Tower as the symbol of his enterprise, ratifying the identification of luxury dolls with Paris as metropolis. Life imitated art in this dispute. On stage in Offenbach's *Tales of Hoffman*, 1881, a dollmaker and his supplier of eyes quarrelled over the rights to the doll Olympia and the profits that she would generate for her manufacturer (Taylor 2000: 62–3).

The intense cult of the doll's trousseau and the shopping for extra items seemed to disappear from the 1880s onwards. By the 1890s, bébés were sold in department stores and advertised widely through illustrated catalogues. Promotional catalogues for New Year's gifts became a focal point of the yearly cycle for major French retailers. Department stores had become the most substantial customers for bébés at the end of the nineteenth century. Some companies, notably Jumeau and Denameur, made bébés especially to order. These dolls were marketed under the name of the commissioning store rather than the maker, dressed in chemises and packaged in designs exclusive to each store. This is a different level of trade to the boutiques of 1860s Paris. As well as the massmarket department stores, more exclusive toy and doll sellers whose names are found on bébés include Au Nain Bleu and Simonne.

Fashion and Aesthetics: Placing the Bébé in the Symbolic Order

When fashion is read as a language of representation and meaning, the bébé demands attention as an out-of-the-ordinary vision of the feminine, enriched by the intense scrutiny of women in Third Republic France. The bébé reifies women as commodities and signs of the 'beautiful', in the capitalist era: an intense schematisation of the female image as fascinating as that expressed through the art of Rossetti, Burne-Jones, Leighton, Tissot and many contemporaries. When this overarching, obsessive sense of 'beauty' is materialised as a childlike doll, woman per se becomes even more lightly weighted in representational content, beyond her function of radiating supreme, compelling beauty, than she is in the narrow hothouse world of nineteenth-century art. Woman's emblematic sexual status as painted temptress in fine arts imagery is reduced and contained by the doll format.

The bébé emphasises the ironies inherent in nineteenth-century attitudes to small girls, especially the simultaneous contradictory discourses of purity and erotic fantasy. If one claims that the Victorian era explicitly sexualised the image of the 'pure' female child that it consciously created and circulated (Kociumbas 1999: 117), even whilst avowing the primacy of its definition of the child as 'innocent', the French bébé reiterates that artistic fetishisation of the child that threads through nineteenth-century art. A wide range of artists, both male and female, emphasise the sexual elements of the elaborate 1870s and 1880s fashions for girls, imaging pre-pubescent girls wearing elaborate frocks, sometimes in crisp white cotton, sometimes in coloured fabrics, frequently matched by elaborate bonnets above long, lanky black-stockinged legs. Girls are frequently posed to reveal drawers and petticoats. Images of prematurely mature, erotic girlhood are found in the work of Mary Cassatt, James Tissot and John Singer Sergeant, amongst many others in the 1870 to 1890 period.

With stockier legs and longer skirts than the painted representations, the bébé used different erotic devices and zones, most notably the meltingly beautiful face with its intense gaze and large eyes to draw attention to the ideal image of the young child as 'beautiful', as well as the fine details of dress and millinery. Bru particularly favoured deep, invitingly parted lips and graceful hands and arms – like the legs of Tissot's girls, prematurely shapely – providing a promise of the woman-to-be in the child of the present. Whilst the doll body is more chunky and immature, some French advertising graphics represent the doll as an alluring girl-woman. A doll advertisement published by the Printemps department store in 1901 (Coleman et al. 1986: 118) and Jumeau booklets are notable examples. The booklet of 1885 entitled *L'Industrie Poetique* (Theimer and Theriault 1994: 102) not only eroticises the swooning doll-child, but also avoids drawing her with joints or any stiffness of pose, thus making her indistinguishable in her lithe form from her living owner. The doll is an exact reduction of her owner. In one illustration from this publication shapely young girls in high fashion dance around a painting of the Jumeau factory. A trade card, produced for Bru in the late 1880s (Theimer 1991: 123), not only shows the dolls as living girls, with short dresses, shapely legs and no joints, but also includes one of their products herself carrying a doubly reduced infant nursing doll. Worked by pneumatic pressure, this nursing doll that sucked fluids from a bottle was one of the Bru company's exclusive lines.

In 1903 British-Australian artist Mortimer Menpes, at various times colleague and rival to James McNeill Whistler, wrote and illustrated, with his wife Dorothy, a book about children of various nations. The Menpes couple regarded the modern sexualisation of the child as tainted and dangerous. However they piously identi-fied such sexually alert children as essentially alien to the British spirit, but entirely typical of France. A French child, elegant and knowing, was hardly a child; everything she did was aimed to the final end of self-display. This performance of high fashion amongst young children indicated the aberrant nature of French concepts of girlhood, as did the French mother's prudent segregation of girls and boys in the neighbourhood, lest a girl make friendships with future sexual and dynastic complications amongst social inferiors (Menpes and Menpes 1903: 54–5). British antique dealer and doll historian Constance Eileen King cogently linked the Menpes' stigmatisation of the sophisticated child-woman favoured by French high society to the bébé (King 1983: 92). Dorothy and Mortimer Menpes dissembled when they ascribed this knowing overwriting of 'childhood' solely to the 'French'; it appeared as a widespread erotic trope throughout European and English-speaking societies in the late-nineteenth and early-twentieth centuries. The Menpes' text indicates that anxieties about the overly mature choices presented to girls by Barbie or 'inappropriately' mature and decorative lingerie have a pre-history suffused with racist prurience.

Late-nineteenth-century female vaudeville entertainers often performed in childlike costumes to intermingle girlishness and sexual display. Whilst Franco-American revue star (of disavowed Polish-Jewish origins) Anna Held was claimed to be a living copy of a Bébé Jumeau, the Barrington Sisters, an American troupe, were extremely successful on the European variety and revue stage in the 1890s. Their image centred upon little-girl style dresses and bonnets in performance. Around 1895 several posters and lithographs by Toulouse-Lautrec featured May Belfort in stage dress of a high-waisted 'Kate Greenway' girl's dress and lacy bonnet. Fin de siècle cabaret and music hall witnessed a plethora of pseudo-infantile acts performed by grown women such as skipping-rope dancers, skirt dancers or singers of popular songs. In childish personae adults performed titles such as 'I Don't Want to Play in Your Yard', 'Won't You Come and Play With Me?', 'Do You Want to See My Pussy?' or 'Daddy Would Not Buy Me a Bow Wow' on the English and European stage. Such performers often affected a sophisticated pastiche of girls' fashions. A German postcard (see Figure 4.4) poses a young woman in pseudo-juvenile bonnet and short skirt, even a child's jewellery, as understood at that period – a Nellie Stewart bangle and a heart-shaped locket. These signifiers of childhood are combined with dress elements bearing a distinct erotic charge – a décolletage, high-heeled shoes, and stockings rolled below the knees. The model holds a bisque doll, as further sign of her playful, pseudo-child identity. The implication of late-nineteenth-century French dolls in this conscious and knowing discourse indicates that dolls can have an affinity to the complex messages projected by fashion.

The bébé is not only about Victorian sexual hypocrisy. She offers fashion historians an unparalleled source of information about the 'look' and character of nineteenth-century French couture, beyond the coloured engraving. Whereas in the

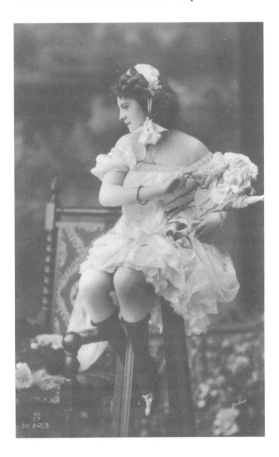

Figure 4.4 Hand-tinted postcard showing woman with doll by Gerlach, German early-1900s.

twentieth century major designers' styles and tastes can be easily distinguished from those of their peers and discussed as historical and cultural entities, with the possible exception of Worth and a handful of contemporaries, 'house style' or handwork traits for many renowned names of nineteenth-century Paris are rarely pinpointed. Few curators have followed Elizabeth Coleman's analysis of named nineteenth-century designers' oeuvres, as individual entities (E.A. Coleman 1989: 7). Valerie Steele suggests that 'by and large the names of these nineteenth-century couturières have been forgotten . . . obliterated by the spectacular rise of the male couturiers' (1991: 23). In this information void the bébé tells us much about the physicality of nineteenth-century French couture such as details of accessorising, including gloves and hosiery, or understanding of accepted colour palettes. She is particularly informative around the relationship of millinery to dress. Long before couture's golden era in the twentieth century, the bébé demonstrates the tactile and sculptural qualities that high-level French fashion production could achieve even in the nineteenth century.

The bébé provides particularly vivid information regarding the last quarter of the nineteenth century, especially the 1880s. As in the 1950s, during the 1880s French couture excelled in elaboration of cut and executional precision, even measured against its own expected high standards. Couture dresses of the 1880s maximised opportunities for bravura detailing on a number of fronts: the sculptural qualities of drape and construction, the tactile qualities of contrasting materials and weaves – elaborate jacquard brocades against satins, silk against velvet, the intense precision of finishing, pleating, cording, piping, braids and passementeries, and the emotional and dramatic language of colour, dark against light, unusual mixtures of hues. All this is to be found in bébés wearing the most formal level of professionally produced outfits.

By the mid-1890s the signifiers of style and taste in French children's dressing shifted and the dressing of bébés also changed. In the 1880s, dolls wore adult-like garments in rich fabrics and complex cut and design. Although there were some slight modifications of form such as shorter skirts following nineteenth-century dress codes that acknowledged children's need for greater informality and freedom, these dolls' rich clothes reflected the basic strategy of imitating adult clothes that had inspired upper-class childrenswear for centuries. In the early-1900s, whitewear seems to have become ubiquitous in French girlswear as a signifier of elegance and status. Many turn-of-the-century French photographs and postcards of girls and dolls show such dresses on doll and child alike. These flimsy cotton, muslin, voile and net garments, of course, implied the presence of servants to launder, starch and iron, speaking, as much as the recently fashionable brocades and satins, of class and wealth. '[T]hus one could demonstrate that one was a lady without anything that is normally called showiness' (Moore 1949: 148). However, this new aesthetic limited the range of materials for dolls' dressmaking and offered fewer 'crossover' opportunities into adultwear. Many later French dolls, from the 1890s onwards wear middle-class frocks, cotton 'school dresses' in plain colours and tartans, and the standard 'mariner' suits or sailor suits. French companies issued dolls in simple chemises for home dressing, or in more humble cotton dresses, throughout the 1890s, and many French dolls clearly wear home-made clothes.

If we accept that one of the pleasures offered by fashion is its irrationality, its surrealist promise and ability to confront and confound those who demand the logical and orderly in the semiotic messages around their lives, then the bébé is a supremely fashionable item, in the folly of her extraordinary self-presentation and female image. If fashion and surrealism are deemed to have cogent links (Martin 1987: 217–25), if the female causes especial problems for the Surrealists (Caws 1997: 35–7; Kuenzli 1995: 17–26), then the bébé as *faux* feminine, as impossibly stereotyped feminine, becomes a quintessential player in the system of fashion. The bébé has appeared rarely in the wider culture of surrealism and twentieth-century art, unlike the store mannequin and the puppet, who were assigned a place in avant-garde twentieth-century culture. The bébé is surely the quintessential *femme-enfant* of surrealist fantasy.

Only Hans Bellmer seems to have capitalised upon the bébé's presence, indicated through the ball-jointed dolls' bodies, which he constantly photographed and referenced throughout the 1930s and later. Indeed our understanding of Bellmer's aesthetic is diminished without knowledge of the format and construction of contemporary dolls. Bellmer responded to one aspect of the bébé: her role as bearer of male voyeurism and sexual predatoriness. Bellmer may also have responded to German dolls as much as the French bébé. He grew up and worked in Germany and his dolls reference young relatives and cousins. Some early drawings of dolls (Taylor 2000: 36–9, 42) clearly depict German-produced dolls. However in terms of early-twentieth-century dolls, all roads, in effect, lead to Paris. German ball-jointed dolls were direct imitations of the bébé, as the composition-bodied, ball-jointed, bisque-headed doll was a French development. This body format was patented in 1861 by Simon-Auguste Brouillet, but only put into effective commercial realisation by the Schmitt and Steiner companies around 1875. The Jumeau bébé followed around 1876 (Theimer and Theriault 1994: 72–4).

Mirka Mora, the French-Australian artist, who trained as an actress and experimented as an artist in Paris after the Second World War before emigrating to Australia, responded to the bébé's surrealist potential. When Mora gained fame after migration to Australia, she was identified in the media as an important collector of French dolls as well as an artist. 'For many years she has been collecting dolls, often paying a *lot* of money – and her *last* money – for a doll' (Beier 1980: 58). It was claimed that she first grew to know the iconic French dolls as a child in Paris in the 1930s, when her father, an antique dealer, would look out for old porcelain dolls on her behalf. In 1971, she boasted that she would never part with her Jumeau doll, even though she was offered the then-immense sum of five hundred Australian dollars (Ellis 1971: 29). The bébé's shadow appears across Mora's art, informing her characteristic big-eyed stylisation of figures and faces. Mora was frequently photographed amongst both her art and her dolls, as testament to her identity as Surrealist.

The reputation and charisma of the nineteenth-century French doll was established not by artists but by doll-collectors. During the 1940s and 1950s, American collectors assumed that French dolls had been dressed by the couture houses of their era, perhaps influenced by the high profile of current French designers in popular consciousness or perhaps confusing the dolls with the recent 1946 showing of the Théâtre de la Mode, a collection of miniature couture fashions, that found a permanent home in the United States. In her editorial comments to a Jumeau advertising book Nina S. Davies specifically refutes this North American belief (Cusset 1957: 8–9). John Noble documents a myth circulated by mid-twentieth-century North American doll collectors that 'a certain dolls' dressmaker of Paris held a licence from the House of Worth, permitting fourteen model dresses to be copied, in dolls' sizes every year'. This story forms part of the 'legacy of tantalizing legends' with 'no factual basis for them' from 'an earlier generation of doll collectors' (Noble 1999: 12). It could also be counted as part of the crossover between couture and popular consumption of fashion articulated by dolls.

The bébé links to a number of stereotyped images that represented 'France' for the non-French in the 1950s and early-1960s: the circus, the mountebank, the sideshow, the puppet, the harlequin, the streetside flower seller, Gavroche – the street urchin. Many of these stereotypes were repeated from popular musical comedies and films such as *Carnival*, 1961, *Lili*, 1953 (both based upon two short fictional works by Paul Gallico: *The Man Who Hated People*, 1950 and its later revision the *Love of Seven Dolls*, 1954) or *An American in Paris*, 1951, and from many examples in two dimensions, graphic and textile design to the big-eyed children prints which became such a popular souvenir of Paris. These signs of 'France' relate to imagery by major twentieth-century artists, for example the more approachable and illustrative works of Picasso in his blue and rose periods or his neoclassical works of the 1915–1930 period. Other frequently seen design elements reference the work of Manet, Renoir and Degas, stripped of their more acidic comments upon social and sexual life. These codified images of 'France' are replicated ad nauseum throughout all levels of fashion publicity and photography in the 1950s. Another cultural referent is the film *Gigi*, 1958. When Leslie Caron appears first as a schoolgirl in a checked dress and large straw hat, she wears the archetypal dress of a later French bébé. As an adult-figured young woman dressed down in child-like drag, Caron embodies the Menpes' stereotyped, sexualised French child of the turn of the century. Images of Audrey Hepburn in the 1951 Broadway stage version of *Gigi* also present a mature young woman wearing a child's mariner dress. This intermingling of adult and child female image was, as noted, frequently seen on the late-nineteenth-century stage.

As the bébé is a child, she expresses the symbolic importance that the child – as natural, unspoiled intellect – carries in Enlightenment value systems as foil to the masculine, developed intellect. The child is a tabula rasa, and can be developed with appropriate guidance into an Enlightenment mind or a docile, attentive breeder of future Enlightenment minds, or the infantry men so necessary for the conflict of the modern nation-state. A child indicates the status of women, children and coloured peoples in Enlightenment discourse, and confirms the right-to-rule accorded to the intellectual by his status. Such a strange, perverted and over-the-top child as the bébé, who is *unheimlich* and hardly-to-be-believed, reflects profound social changes after the Franco-Prussian war, especially in the strongly contested position of women in public and cultural life in the Third Republic. Albert Boime suggests that women began to symbolise particularly new and urgent anxieties in relation to the French state. The feminine highlighted the overturning of expected order during the siege of Paris, and therefore the control/supervision of the feminine indicated a return of civil authority and autonomy in French society (Boime 1995: 89-94, 116–17). Likewise, Valerie Steele indicates how a trousered woman, seen in an engraving of a Paris street during the siege of Paris, symbolised the disruptions the siege caused to the expected social fabric (1999: 166–7). Thus debates around the registration and regulation of prostitutes were not simply about public health or the efficient organisation of sexual commerce, but an indicative metaphor for the deep-seated, but hard-to-promulgate, need to surveil all women.

Women represented the feminised weakness of Napoleon III's regime, as well as the feminine state of subjection and despoliation, especially the sense of the permeability of borders, during the German occupation. Empress Eugénie, whose beauty was, as we have seen, replicated by the Parisienne dolls, was regarded by intellectuals as a symbol of the weakness of the Second Empire and the improper order of feminine influence over the male domain of public and political life (Dolan 1994: 24–5). The bébé turns woman as troubling symbol of disorder and defeat into a charming and ingratiating child-dependant. In early sources, Emile-Louis Jumeau was imaged as a hero, capable of controlling aberrant women, from badly behaved daughters of good families to fallen women, through his dolls (Peers 1997: 67).

Because her charms are far less discreet than those of the Parisienne, her essentialised function of pleasing the male eye may lead one to underestimate the cultural message of the bébé. Certainly Emile-Louis Jumeau had a complex psychological relationship to his own dolls that collector literature entirely overlooks.

> As for my disposition, it is of the sweetest. Possessed of matchless philosophy my placidness is unbounded. You may according to the impulse of the moment or your fancy, caress or flog me, kiss or strike me, hold me topsy turvey, or dash me to the ground; I shall smile none the less . . . (Anon c.1880: np)

This desire for an easy, uncomplicated relationship with women was not solely a personal whim for Jumeau. The desire for a limpid, straightforward woman, who asserted no freewill, also indicates woman's problematical nature to the Third Republic as image and metaphor. A disorderly woman or a woman out of control indicated a similar loss of control or order in the public sphere. Hollis Clayson suggests that not only erotic obsession made the prostitute a central figure in French high-cultural imaging in the late-nineteenth century, but prostitution highlighted the understanding that modern social relationships were 'more and more frozen in the form of the commodity' (Clayson 1991: 9). The doll herself abstracted human relations and emphasised the monetary exchange in transactions between adult males even more than the prostitute (Peers 1997: 72–6).

> He saw them in all the shops for novelties and toys unceasingly provoking the admiration of visitors . . . he contemplated them in their naive splendour, with their beautiful blond or brunette hair, their large expressive eyes, their arms extended to be kissed, their beautiful dresses in Marquise style, their beautiful hats in today's fashion . . . (Paul Laure 'Le Bébé Jumeau et le Magnitisme', article from unidentified Parisian newspaper, 3 December 1887; qtd Theimer and Theriault 1994: 110)

In this short story the Jumeau dolls, whom the *flâneur* sees all about the city of Paris, lead an unsuspecting Parisian gentleman – who is seeking to understand why his daughter cried when *Petit Noel* did not bring a Bébé Jumeau – not to a brothel, but to a factory where 'in perfect order . . . excellent working men and women make all the pieces of Bébé Jumeau'. The visibility of women in the modern city is acknowledged, for the doll is as present as the prostitute in the new commercial spaces, but the bébé ultimately upholds orderly social and industrial relations, unlike the total disintegration of public order during the siege of Paris.

Fashion and self-presentation facilitate Bébé Jumeau's upholding of the social norms, rather than indicating female folly and frivolity's potential to undermine male order and progress. The *flâneur* was gratified by the self-presentation of the dolls whom he saw across the city. 'Oh! he thought, toys are progressing along with the century. They have become elegant, fine, spiritual: thanks to Bébé Jumeau they refine the taste of our young girls, they teach them grace of demeanour, the charms of costume . . .' (qtd Theimer and Theriault 1994: 110). The prostitute was a potent symbol in modern France, 'emblematic of the place of women in the dominant regime of visual representation of women in the west in the modern period' (Clayson 1991: 9). In late-nineteenth-century Paris, the doll clearly also shared this task of negotiating the position of women and of modern life.

In texts Bébé Jumeau provided even more fundamental reassurances. Much of the advertising copy around her proclaims her victory over the German doll. This victory is usually defined in terms of nationalism: that the French bébé must prevail over the German doll, due to her grace and superior style, and, above all, her greater appeal to aesthetics and the eye. In one example of Jumeau advertising copy, however, German identity is written as abjectivity, animalism and the human body's ultimate vulnerability and susceptibility to penetration. The citizen's body threatens to manifest itself as equally fragile and permeable as the nation proved to be when the Prussians and other German armies swarmed over France in 1870. Rather than the order and control promised by the beautiful, perfected French doll, German dolls emphasised the essentially weak physicality of the body, especially under conditions of stress, its 'meagreness', its 'stench', its animalistic moans.

These words are enough to terrify those frightened German babies. They are ugly and ridiculous enough, those German dolls with their stupid faces of wax-over-composition, their goggle eyes, and their meagre straw bodies. I would rather be mute than have an animal's sound come out of my chest. I am not a fighter young Miss, but I can assure you that when the day happens that I come face to face with one of them, I will break her cardboard body as if it were glass, with its stench of candle grease and wax. I am of course a true French bébé! (qtd Melger 1997: 40–41)

Bébé Jumeau's elegance is neither vanity nor self-indulgence but a brave defence against mortality and atrophy. Two different models of Jumeau bébés are actually saviours of France in female drag. The Bébé Triste, designed by Carrier-Belleuse, is modelled after Bosio's 1824 sculpture of the young King Henri IV, and Bébé Français is a portrait of the Duc de Bordeaux, the chief Bourbon claimant after the 1830 Revolution. The Duc was proclaimed as Henri V, but refused to reign under the republican *tricouleur*. Jumeau was definitely not a Bonapartist. Many of his bébés stand on Napoleonic bees imprinted on the soles of their shoes, thus enacting an insult that is traditional in many cultures.

The extravagant and finely made dresses worn by the top level of bébés, highlight their invisibility in present-day fashion consumption. Could one conceive of a modern child's doll, dressed to the standard expected of seasonal couture collections, an iconic showpiece of Baby Dior or Junior Gaultier? Why did the bébé disappear? Why have childhood and high fashion clearly parted company? Why did a significant subsection of the Paris couture industry, the luxury doll trade, disappear by the late-1890s? The Jumeau company was constantly likened to couture houses by its contemporaries. Collectors' literature provides no clear answer.

Later in the 1890s the Parisian doll trade struggled against cheaper German imports, represented by the Eden Bébé. The doll sold well, as she was cheaper than French dolls and appeared to advantage in the department stores which were becoming the new focus of doll retailing. Though sold in their thousands throughout the 1890s, in France and elsewhere, Eden Bébés were actually German dolls packaged and presented to appear like French dolls. They were made by Fleischmann and Bloedel, a German company which François Theimer claims (1991: 145) appears to have been formed with the express intention of making a corporate raid on the French doll industry. Much of the documentation around the Fleischmann and Bloedel company has been written from the perspective of those companies damaged and bankrupted by its actions. Looking at them now, it seems strange that a French-sounding name and a lower price could allow these ordinary dolls to 'pass' as French dolls so frequently that the local industry was destabilised and the esteemed manufacturers witnessed a rapid drop in their profits during the 1890s.

A detailed and relatively mature discussion of the demise of the French doll industry was written by Jeanne Doin for the *Gazette des Beaux Arts*. She indicates that good quality German porcelain heads cost about a quarter of the price of similar French heads. The German companies shipped promptly and efficiently and offered ample facilities for credit (Doin 1916: 434; von Boehn 1966: 164–5). In 1915 it was noted that, whilst patriotic manufacturers may have produced dolls from French components, French domestic buyers would not accept the more expensive native product (d'Avenel 1915: 345). Therefore French customers seeking cheaper product facilitated German dominance. Even Emile-Louis Jumeau imported some heads with both open- and closed-mouths from the German Simon and Halbig firm in the 1890s,[2] although no accessible written information indicates how he could have justified this action in light of his publicly stated antipathy to German dolls in his promotional material.

If much doll-collector literature casts the defeat of the bébé as a precursor to the two World Wars and German territorial and military ambitions, the course of twentieth-century political and military history is perhaps inappropriately inserted into the nineteenth-century toy trade. Some see Fleischmann and Bloedel, and the later SFBJ, as a German plot to sink the French doll industry (Theimer 1991: 145; Theimer and Theriault 1994: 178, 180, 183). British researcher June Jackson noted that Salomon Fleischmann was married to a Frenchwoman and lived in Paris (Jackson 2001). Fleischmann's descendants remained involved with the SFBJ company for half a century (Coleman et al. 1986: 1092), and his children in turn married into French families. If Fleischmann were integrated into French social and familial life, what was the advantage for him of working on behalf of German imperial economic interests? If Fleischmann and Bloedel have been claimed as a metaphor for Pan-Germanism, German militarism and racism could the evidence be read differently to suggest that Fleischmann and Bloedel were an avatar, not of the two World Wars but of later European cross-border economic cooperation? If the intention was to undermine the French doll industry and facilitate German exports, why did Fleischmann and Bloedel set up a cartel, the SFBJ, which sold successfully against Germany in the French domestic market, the French colonial market, Australia and South America (Coleman et al. 1970: 586, 588)?

Certainly the SFBJ was not the only conglomerate to be formed out of individual French companies c.1900. Barbara Day, writing for Dorothy McGonagle's history of Steiner dolls, records that manufacturers of tin and clockwork toys and manufacturers of board games formed consortiums in France at the same period. Smaller, less solvent firms were swallowed and disappeared (McGonagle 1988: 17). Day suggests that the financial difficulties of the Parisian doll firms were part of a general downturn in French business. During the 1870s and 1880s small-scale manufacturing could be supported by hard work, good ideas and quality product; by the 1890s solvent and viable manufacturers had to be 'part of a large system'

(1998: 16) with factories rather than ateliers, to survive. However the adult couture trade did not succumb to this economic slump, though it was already, by the 1890s, thoroughly integrated into the national economy. French couture maintained its reputation internationally amongst its customers. Its authority and appeal never diminished. One early French commentator (d'Avenel 1915: 344) suggests that the McKinley tariff laws of the early-1890s shattered the bébé trade that was strongly dependent upon the United States. The French fashion industry was already equally engaged with the North American trade; why did the import of couture garments not also suffer from the rise in excise and charges? If the only failing of Bébé Jumeau was her high price (1915: 344), which finally robbed her of her market share, conversely French couture flourished despite the premium demands it made upon its clients' purses.

An independent commentator on the French doll trade, Albert Blake Dick, provides an interesting and detached commentary on the actual nature of the doll industry in Paris in the late-1880s. Dick was touring Europe in 1889 collecting samples and making contacts to assist in Thomas Alva Edison's attempt to develop and manufacture a talking doll. He sent reports back in letters now stored at Edison National Historic Site. Approaching French dolls from neither an aesthetic nor a nationalist point of view, he provides a more sober assessment of the strengths and many weaknesses of the industry as a whole.

> I have just about concluded my investigation of the doll trade in Paris, and contrary to my first impression, I have found it confined principally to one concern doing a business of over 300,000 dolls annually.
>
> There are twelve dollmakers in this city, but excepting the business done by M.Jumeau above referred to, all are in my estimation doing a very light business. As a class they are not strong financially, and are to be found mostly in lofts located in cheap districts and, like many other businesses conducted here, bear the stamp of being run on 'hand to mouth' principles.
>
> Jumeau is represented as the only manufacturer in France who makes every part of the dolls that he sells, from the wigs to the soles of the shoes . . . [He] is also strong financially . . .
>
> His factories are large, and he employs over 1000 hands, mostly women and girls. (qtd Wood 2002: 144)

Dick's letter backs up Barbara Day's suggestion that the French doll and toy industry was financially vulnerable and could not survive the transition from handmade to industrial production.

And why the massive drop in production standard? This rapid loss of quality cannot be blamed on the German doll industry. In the early-1900s many German manufacturers easily exceeded SFBJ products in quality. There were enough skilled French advisors around the SFBJ to assist the new entity, which also had access to both factories and skilled workforces of companies such as Jumeau. The Jumeau daughters remained on the SFBJ board until the 1950s. The pragmatic Paul Eugene Girard, who had run down standards at the house of Bru, was closely associated with the SFBJ. Two generations of his descendants worked for the firm. The loss of quality can be clearly read after he assumed management at Bru. Perhaps he did the same with the SFBJ?

Did the bébé herself lose favour? Had tastes changed so rapidly that there was no place for her in the twentieth century except when extreme circumstances of war and politics demanded that the skills and vision of the French doll industry were revived? Why did the French – seemingly overnight – lose all interest in an effective and popular channel for communicating the uniqueness and status of French fashion? The French wholeheartedly embraced innovations in fashion and marketing throughout the twentieth century and into the twenty-first. Newer means of communicating stylistic change and innovation than the doll, such as photo-gravure and the cinema newsreel, adopted by the fashion industry did not make fashion dolls disappear. High fashion dolls again became extremely popular in North America during the 1950s when all of the key information media for fashion promotion deployed in the second half of the twentieth century were already flourishing, with the exception of internet-based systems of information delivery. Were definitions of childhood changing? Was fashion seen as more appropriate for an adult woman than a child? Was the child's 'naturalness' pitched against the artificiality and corruptive, duplicitous flexibility of fashion? Or could the luxuri-ous, high fashion doll no longer communicate information about its owner's status and consumption, and therefore did tastemaking and fashion validate other indices of cultural awareness leaving the doll to the nursery? Did production standards fall when the doll was relegated to the child's world? Doll collectors have never posed these questions and material answering these questions has never been circulated in collectors' publications. At least one researcher, Barbara Day, admits that evidence about the decline of one French company is hard to locate, and, therefore, drawing conclusions from such an information void is impossible (qtd McGonagle 1988: 17–18).

One clear difference between the dollmarket at c.1880 and c.1900, which made the bébé less welcome in the marketplace, was the emerging psychological and medical surveillance of the individual and the domestic environment. Was Sig-mund Freud rather than Fleischmann and Bloedel responsible for the bébé's demise?

–5–

Decline of the French Doll Industry and the Fate of the Fashionable Doll During the Twentieth Century

As French cultural theorist Roland Barthes writes, 'French toys always mean something, and this something is always entirely socialised, constituted by the myths or the techniques of modern adult life'. He continues, 'the fact that French toys literally prefigure the world of adult functions obviously can not but prepare the child to accept them all, by constituting for him, even before he can think of it, the alibi of Nature which has at all times created soldiers, postmen and Vespas.' Whether French or American, toys convey a great deal about how adults wish children to grow up, and as Barthes observes, toys prepare us for the roles we wish children to think of as 'natural'. What roles do we wish girls to grow up and assume are 'natural'?

Sherrie A. Inness 'Barbie Gets a Bum Rap' (1999: 181)

The Stigmatisation of the Fashion Doll

The demise of the French doll industry remains under documented beyond the clear trajectory of cost cutting and lowering of standards amongst makers during the 1890s, and the emergence of the imported Fleischmann and Bloedel dolls as key players in the French domestic market. Secondary literature tends to lack trade and marketplace statistics and invokes emotive nationalist issues. Yet French dollmaking during the late-1890s not only suffered economic collapse, but also a failure of design initiative. Theimer inferred that the last director of the Bru company, Paul Girard, did not have the aesthetic discrimination of the previous directors (1991: 114–21, 131–6). Examination of later Bru dolls upholds Theimer's judgement. There are few parallels in twentieth-century design history to the decline of the French doll. Evolving technologies and patterns of consumption and promotion have tended to encourage a trajectory of aesthetic and experimental expansion in modern design and applied art products. With dolls not merely did a design product disappear, but also the values that drove it. In other media, from glass and ceramics to fashion, French design in the first decades of the twentieth century was outstanding and found favour with discriminating customers internationally. Whereas French Haute Couture was an esteemed design medium throughout the twentieth century, the cultural trajectories of French dollmaking and fashion over the past century are obviously different. Historical and political events rather than the aesthetic savvy of dollmaking allowed the two disciplines to occasionally merge.

By 1900 German dollmakers monopolised all levels of the international doll trade. The high end of the German doll industry always claimed to be less vulgar or baroque than the French dolls. The cheaper end of German doll production simply undercut the prices of French manufacturers, relying upon the public to not be particularly alert to the differences in style or quality between French and German dolls. Emile-Louis Jumeau saw differences in quality of design and production between the two nations' doll industries as crucial to both the identity of his product and to his nation's reputation. This difference between French and German product was performed through the superior appearance of his dolls but their beauty also expressed a national urgency. French dolls were not only outstanding in looks and dress, but they also represented a major source of export income and expressed the superiority of the French cause and spirit. However, the buying public did not share Jumeau's discrimination. Ironically, both domestic and overseas customers seemed to be indifferent to these matters which were so crucial for Jumeau. Economic competition prompted the French doll to be altered so much that she became a mere poor-quality imitation of the German doll.

German dolls were only about 'fashion' to the extent that the *geistlich,* eternal spirituality of the high-end German doll, and the practical price cutting at the low end of the market, together 'defeated' the luxury French doll. Thus the close connections between dolls and fashion were sundered early in the twentieth century. German dolls set the character doll, a doll moulded to express a portrait-like realism of emotion, with a humanist *gravitas* or a whimsical sense of fun against the supposed vapidity of the fashion doll. Undoubtedly the first priority of the German industry was opportunistic: to imitate the admired French production and deliver it at a cheaper pricepoint to gain orders. However, turn-of-the-century psychology and sociology further placed German doll companies in a secure economic position. New attitudes towards dolls, maternity and the scrutiny of the female child favoured the German approach, which highlighted the doll as an object for training girls in domestic and mothering responsibilities rather than in consuming fashion. Explicit ideologies around dolls followed in the wake of increasing psychological and psychiatric surveillance of everyday life by 'experts' and these ideologies favoured German over French dolls.

From early-twentieth-century Germany there emerged a movement to create a 'reformed' doll. The targets of these reforms were fashionable French dolls or German dolls that, influenced by the French approach to dollmaking, presented an idealised, elaborate vision of femininity. Politically, to some degree, this reform had a left-wing, liberative promise. The movement started in the artistic Sezessions, progressively minded artists' groups and the handcraft guilds, most notably the Munich Art Workers' Guild, and spread to other cities including Berlin, Dresden and Karlsruhe (von Boehn 1966: 178). The doll reform movement emerged from the broad currency of William Morris's ideas in Germany in the context of the general design reform of German industrial products in the early 1900s that in turn would lead in the post-1918 era to the Bauhaus. Concurrently, vocabularies of systematic educational and psychological theories were transforming public health discourses of childhood development. The doll came under professional scrutiny. No longer were dolls to be 'unnatural objects' with a 'superabundance of all too concrete details' (von Boehn 1966: 177), but they were to be well made and cultivate an appropriately healthy state of mind in their owners. Dolls were targets of social welfare reforms similar to those that sought to regulate household life, especially of lower-class citizens in the emerging twentieth-century nation-states, by officially instituting 'healthier' options and models. Even as early as 1887 German opinion expressed anxieties about the baroque quality of elaborate French dolls, suggesting that they were beyond the needs or comprehension of a child, as evidenced by a comment traced by Stuart Holbrook in the *Berliner Zeitung* of that year (qtd Holbrook 1990: 82).

In early-twentieth-century texts strong nationalist paradigms surface in the wording of the abuse directed against the French doll, which was seen as shallow, untrustworthy and manipulative. 'The French never spare themselves self praise . . . only rarely are French fashions real inventions of Paris, usually they come from other sources' (von Boehn 1966: 134). Criticism of French fashion and the febrility of content in French design have a Pan-Germanist resonance. Max von Boehn quoted a number of contemporary German opinions around anxieties about the fashionable – therefore French – doll (1966: 175–7).

Late-nineteenth-century German anxieties about the correct socialisation of girl children through dolls not only were shared by both right- and left-wing elements of the Second Reich, but have survived to operate in the denunciations of Barbie on similar terms in the very different socio-political context of the postwar democracies. For some, Barbie simultaneously promotes capitalism and a shallow, sensualised vision of the female body. These denunciations of Barbie centre on an absurdist reduction of both fashion and female agency to a series of evil mask-like caricatures, which denies the complex series of strategies that surround both fashion and women's gesture as consumer. Women's pleasure and agency within the discourse of fashion is evaded.

Generally, paradigmatic feminist anxieties about Barbie and paradigmatic feminist anxieties about fashion strongly overlap. Valerie Steele identifies a history of major feminist thinkers such as de Beauvoir and Friedan who, in the mid-twentieth century, objected to high fashion (1991: 119). Stella Bruzzi outlines this history of second-wave feminist anxieties around fashion in further detail (1997:

121–24, 126–7). Bruzzi suggests that for feminists 'the vicissitudes of female dress ultimately undermine the woman and render her subservient to (and the victim of) the man who retains his iconographic stability' (Bruzzi 1997: 120). Ironically the fashion-based signifiers of the trope of the modern cinematic femme fatale– short skirts, high heels, long legs, blonde hair, 'boldly coloured' clothes that Bruzzi identifies (1997: 126–9, 135–7, 139–40) – could also describe the classic pinkbox Barbie from 1977 onwards. Bruzzi consciously inverts the second-wave feminist argument regarding fashion to suggest that in late-twentieth-century films, the seductively, quintessentially, femininely dressed woman can exert a significant and transgressive power over conventional and domestic characters or male weakness. Likewise M.G. Lord also demonstrates that a polyvalent feminist power exists in that which second-wave feminists reject: Barbie.

Turn-of-the-century denunciations of French dolls had a wide currency through-out many different regimes and cultures. Thus after a 'Russian Toy Congress' in the 1890s passed a resolution protesting 'against the large, elegant French dolls that taught love of dress and suggested luxury', this protest was ratified and circulated to an English-speaking audience in 1897 when cited by influential North American anthropological and psychiatric theorist G. Stanley Hall in his late-nineteenth-century study on dolls (Coleman et al. 1986: 1019). The same protest against French dolls was also quoted in Max von Boehn's history of dolls (1966: 176), which has frequently been used as a key source on doll history. Von Boehn men-tioned the Russian protest in the context of his generalised survey of the modern doll trade in Europe from around the 1880s to the 1920s, and his ratification, written during the Weimar Republic, of the impetus of the German doll reform movement. From the date of the Russian protest in the 1890s, it is clear that luxury French dolls such as the Parisiennes and bébés were targeted by the congress. In particular it was mentioned that the 'large French dolls' condemned by the confer-ence had the 'power of walking, speaking and singing' (von Boehn 1966: 176). There was only one 'singing' doll of the 1890s: Jumeau's Bébé Phonographe, who was the first doll with a recorded voice and a technically viable mechanism that is still operable in some surviving examples. Notably, for a modern reader, and as noted previously, the paradigmatic nature of the protest is the same as that directed so often towards Barbie. Inappropriate dolls foster too strong a 'love of dress' and 'luxury' in growing girls. In current vocabulary the words 'fashion' and 'con-sumerism' may be used, but the parallel nature of the sentiments across the genera-tions is clear.

Ironically, when an Australian academic in 2002 sought to unpick the paradoxes and failure to deliver of the New World Order and post-Soviet Russia, she took protest against fashionable dolls back to Russia a century after the congress's condemnation of fashionable dolls, by selecting as her key metaphor the incon-gruity of the Barbie shop on St Petersburg's Nevsky Prospekt. Fashion in the shape of Barbie is pitted against raw humanity, nurturing values and the need to survive. The pure and acceptable is contrasted to the false and delusional. 'Barbie cares only for fashion and frivolity while the beggars are concerned primarily with food . . . Barbie dresses to portray a style, a carefully fashioned femininity. The beggars heap every scrap they can muster on their weather-assaulted bodies. They are oblivious to fashion' (Varney 2002: 41). This falsehood is defined as 'femininity'; it is seen as 'frivolity' and its key expression is 'fashion'. The concepts of female insufficiency, consumerism, fashion and Barbie are seen as mutually interchangeable; each is a sign of the other and each is to be resisted equally. Conversely the beggars are non-gendered, essentialised, humanist 'everymen' and are concerned with fundamental issues of life, food and shelter rather than styling. The contrast has pietistic and evangelical as much as Marxist overtones. Woman is not only frivolous and superficial, but carries a sort of social cancer in terms of consumerism, capitalism and destabilising the public space '. . . citizenship seemingly without conscience, but ablaze with parties, fashion frenzies and choking levels of consumption' (Varney 2002: 41). Conversely the basic human unit of the left-wing utopia is identified as the beggar, and essentialised as presumed masculine placed in opposition to the error of feminised fashion.

These protests of liberal good taste often carry a deep vein of hypocrisy.

> Many [upper middle-class women] object to [Barbie] on feminist grounds – one hears the familiar 'that body is not in nature' refrain. Then the word bimbo arises. But let a woman talk longer – reassuring her that she is not speaking for attribution – and she'll express her deepest reservation: that 'Barbie is cheap' where the whole idea of 'cheap' is rooted in social hierarchies and economics. (Lord 1994: 183)

Barbie is frequently disavowed by academics, thinkers, elites with a 'Euro-communist' outlook in a wider series of refusals of North America and capitalism that again speak ambiguously about modern life and experience, especially the lived cultural choices of the working classes. Mario Tosa indicates that in rejections of Barbie as a 'pusher . . . for forcibly induced needs' (1998: 114) there is a degree of facileness (1998: 12) when 'the most disparate messages fill every moment of daily life and expectations are piled high, giving voice to the wishes and needs of others . . . All Barbie does is put us in the scene – the preexisting adult world – along with the manias and conventions that have become part of our daily lives' (1998: 115–16). He suggests that because Barbie is an eloquent, adaptive symbol of modern life, those who loathe her, loathe modernity (1998: 9).

> We really ought to ask ourselves how such a simple toy, whose underlying concept is so similar to nineteenth century dolls/mannequins can provoke so much criticism and rage. Perhaps to adults Barbie is the perfect scapegoat, a ubiquitous reminder of a way of life mirrored with discomforting realism. (1998: 9–10)

Such protests of liberal 'good taste' against Barbie are destabilised when the imperial and colonial sources of the definition of the 'correct' or 'appropriate' doll and her correct function in a (female) child's life are revealed.

Doll reform was promoted by competitions and exhibitions in various German cities. The first prototypes to meet with widespread enthusiasm are generally credited to artist Marion Kaulitz and the Munich Art Dolls created by the Art Workers' Guild (D.S. and E.J. Coleman 1997: 70–72). Other artists who designed dolls included Ernst Kirchner, Koloman Moser, Swedish artist Carl Larson and several lesser-known avant-garde German artists, as well as applied art groups such as the Wiener Werkstätte. In the wake of the rapid success of the Munich Art Dolls the commercial toy trade responded. The Kämmer and Reinhardt series of bisque porcelain dolls based upon 'real' children started an immediate trend amongst industrial/commercial manufacturers to emulate the 'Sezession' reformist dolls. However the first series of dolls moulded to look like children in non-idealised moods and vivid expression were Jumeau's *Serie Fantastique* in the 1890s (Theimer and Theriault 1994: 185, 352–72).

Käthe Kruse's cloth dolls were a high-profile response to improving available dolls prior to the First World War. They were regarded as simpler and more holistic than ceramic dolls, therefore they were claimed to express a radical craft ethos, rather than superficial commercialism. Kruse, like Marion Kaulitz, came from an avant-garde background. She was the wife of a professional sculptor and presented her dolls as dissonant with the conventional mainstream culture of Wilhelmine Germany. Today maternalist discourses are generally read as right-wing. However, Kruse's intense focus on motherhood implied a positioning as a challenge to a society in which the individual was repressed, alienated from her basic psychological instincts, in this case it is the female child whose mothering instincts are denied/perverted by the tawdry, artificial dolls that she is given.

> My dolls, particularly the babies, arose from the desire to awaken a feeling that one was holding a real baby in one's arms . . . And the problem of the doll, tantamount to education in maternal feeling, education in womanly act and womanly bliss, perhaps in a better understanding between mother and child, between mother and mother – this whole problem of the doll has certainly sufficient interest in itself. (qtd King 1977: 470)

Kruse's dolls remained as popular and well regarded in the Weimar Republic as they were in both the Imperial and Nazi periods, perhaps they were dolldom's Vicars of Bray. Kruse's dolls particularly demonstrate the duality of 'reformed' dolls. The firm's advertisement in the 1924/26 *Universal Spielwaren Katalog* published by John Hess of Hamburg identified the values behind the Kruse dolls: 'They are washable, soft and unbreakable and they signify: Education to motherliness' (punctuation sic; qtd Bachmann 1985: 361). Doll reform was not only about good product design or replacing the trite and conventional with the well considered, it was also about enabling a girl child to face the future armed with appropriate tools for her appointed role. Concurrently the anti-mass-production, avant-garde arts and crafts values were emphasised in the same paragraph alongside an essentialised image of woman as mother: 'All Käthe Kruse dolls are made entirely of woven stuff, including the heads and are, save for some few machinal [sic] seams are purely hand made . . . The manufacture is under the permanent personal control of Mrs Käthe Kruse' (qtd Bachmann 1985: 361).

The doll reform movement also found a responsive audience in the state and the upper classes. The new style of dolls were bought by royalty including the Kaiserin (D.S. and E.J. Coleman 1997: 70–72). One of the most famous and the first of the 'character dolls' marketed in response to the doll reform initiatives, Kämmer and Reinhardt's first realistic baby doll, was known (especially in English-speaking countries) as the 'Kaiser Baby', as he – and this doll is never regarded or dressed as a 'she' – was erroneously believed to be a portrait of one of Kaiser Wilhelm II's six sons (King 1977: 390). Another realistic German baby doll of the pre-First World War era was associated with German royalty: the 'Baby Stuart' made by Gebrüder Heubach. The Catholic Kings of Bavaria were regarded as an older, more authentic royal house than the German Imperial house of Hohenzollern. Amongst evidence of their mystic *über*-authenticity in regal status was the claim – still current – that the Kings of Bavaria, through marriage to the sole heir of the state of Modena, were the legitimate Kings of England, usurped by Protestants. Indeed where the Kaiser Baby was fiercely masculine in his modelled expression, a credible heir to the *Aussenpolitik* of the Second Reich, the Baby Stuart was equally realistic in his modelling, but pensive, and solemn, a child weighted with a familial inheritance of centuries of regal dignity and medieval religiosity. Forgotten ironic details of German monarchist loyalties are played out in antique doll collections.

The Kaiser Baby identifies the new issues that early-twentieth-century dolls were expected to represent. In this value system fashionable dolls came to be seen as unhealthy or unnatural in relation to essentialised values of childhood, and the baby doll was often pitted against the fashion doll. The Kaiser Baby was perhaps the first baby doll to express something other than a schematised cherub expression, unlike the first Victorian wax babies. His rather fierce, arrogant expression, and the impossibility of cross-dressing him to either gender as desired, as can be done with most antique and modern baby dolls,[1] has probably kept the doll's nickname alive. By settling the baby doll's identity as masculine, this 'realistic', non-tawdry doll reiterates the integration of mothers into the state. The first celebrated 'new born', the Bye-Lo Baby, designed by Grace Storey Putnam in America and made in Germany, dates from 1922, even deeper into the era of Freudian-based maternalist discourses. The model was found in a California public hospital and the artwork sent to German dollmakers by the American wholesaler.

As the quintessential baby the Bye-Lo – no longer the supposed son of an emperor – was eminently a child of the new scientific and medical supervision of childhood. The Bye-Lo Baby also references popular images of capitalism in its nickname the 'Million Dollar Baby', immortalised in a popular song of the period. At Christmas 1922 people queued up in North American toy shops to buy the 'wonder doll' (King 1977: 441).

The most popular interwar baby doll was a German model known in English as 'My Dream Baby': a sweet-faced and pacific persona, but again barely a few days or weeks old and needing to be thoroughly mothered by the modern young girl. The heads were made by the Armand Marseille company and sold to many other companies around the world that assembled the dolls. In Australia ceramic Dream Baby heads from Germany were imported throughout the 1930s right up to the outbreak of the Second World War and assembled with Australian-made bodies and dresses by two different companies, Laurie Cohen and Hoffnungs, both of Sydney (Fainges 1993: 57, 65, 67, 68, 69–70). Complete Dream Babies were also exported internationally from Germany, having been fitted with bodies by various companies. Heads produced at the Armand Marseille factory were purchased by many German dollmakers and the Marseille firm also assembled their own models. The Second World War caused a major crisis when the Dream Babies – more welcomed than most emissaries from the Third Reich – stopped coming.

Thus the cultural image of the ideal baby doll moved from the uncanny, patriotic vision of every girl child bearing/mothering an emperor's son – and thereby rendering up their bodies for imperial glory/service as would their brothers through compulsory military training – to the baby as personal wish-fulfilment and goal (i.e. 'My Dream') and thereby a guardian of woman's psychiatric health/normality. Baby dolls began as idealised angels and cherubs: the soft and passive Victorian wax baby (akin to traditions of wax portraits and funerary effigies seen in Europe from the Renaissance onwards, and the wax Christ Childs from Christmas Crèches) in his or her formal long robes, which implied motherhood as social display, whilst servants did the dirty work amongst the vomit and shit. The trajectory ended with the realism and direct involvement in mothering and homemaking implied by the 'lifelike' infant, who needed to be changed and fed. Scientific realism fixed female children's play identities as mothers. Design and manufacture of dolls followed in the wake of these theories further rendering fashionable lady dolls as aberrant; this position still informs professional and popular attitudes to dolls like Barbie.

> In the 'twenties [rubber] gained an additional cachet from the fact that psychologists attached a great deal of importance to the part played in a child's development by correct 'doll play'. Rubber seemed ideally suited to reproduce a human baby in as lifelike a fashion as possible, and it was now felt that these rubber creations represented a far more healthy force in the child's fantasy world than stiff richly dressed figures of wax or china.

Rubber dolls were especially suitable for bathing, feeding and nappy changing – all the natural functions of a mother towards her baby, which a child might have watched its own mother performing towards a younger brother and sister . . . (Fraser 1964: 106)

Dollmakers themselves exploited these new theories for advertising purposes. In 1924 Effanbee, a New York company, produced a booklet for mothers entitled *The Proper Doll for my Child's Age,* which offered ' a few hints on lessons children learn through doll play' (*Playthings*, August 1924; qtd Coleman et al. 1986: 383).

Compared with Barbie, few academic commentators have expressed qualms about baby dolls and their possible meanings. Sherrie A. Inness however reads a sinister and limiting message from the modern proliferation of baby dolls:

I was surrounded by baby dolls that all conveyed the same message that having a baby is the greatest experience of a woman's life, and every girl should want a baby more than anything else. These dolls did not teach about the importance of travel and adventure; they taught about the importance of maternity and domesticity. They also conveyed the completely unrealistic message that babies are all a woman (or a girl) needs for complete bliss. Lessons like this can lead many girls to have babies while still teenagers, thinking that children are enough to fill someone's life with joy. (Inness 1999: 180)

Knowing baby dolls' origins and the stories behind their manufacture places Inness's personal reaction in a firm social-historical context and problematises the general assumption of the baby doll's beneficence and neutrality. Barbie, ironically, is placed as evil, unnatural and manipulative against the naturalness of the baby doll.

Later in the twentieth century, plastic baby dolls were modelled as genitally complete, and sold with umbilical binding and identity tag, as if the child who received it had recently given birth to it, in a further move to realism in representing babies. More lifelike representation makes baby dolls even more prescriptive. Modern genitally complete baby dolls address motherhood no less insistently than the Victorian initiatives to present girl children with doll infants, augmenting the social and fashion guidance communicated by adult dolls with the homemaker's role. Gendered and complete baby dolls document a psychological 'health', a relaxed and flexible attitude towards sex, but only to a certain degree: adult male dolls intended for children, such as Ken and Action Man, still only display generalised 'bulges'.

M.G. Lord and Erica Rand have identified how sexuality complicates the design and production of male dolls. There was much anxious workshopping of prototypes for Ken in relation to his genitalia. Too small and the male doll would be neutered. As a neutered male figure, Ken would invite contempt for his ambiguous or inadequate gender and be granted only a lowly position in the symbolic hierarchy, but if his genitalia were moulded too large little girls could become pruriently interested in what the 'bulge' represented, or, even worse, they could possibly be frightened out of heterosexuality and motherhood by fears provoked by an overly tumescent Ken (Lord 1994: 49; Rand 1995: 44). If he were presented not with a 'bulge', but with medical textbook directness, Ken could provoke even more distress. The ongoing importance of Freudian theories in the early 1960s, when Ken was being developed, meant that Ken could not sidestep his crucial function of representing heterosexual maleness in a growing girl's universe. Whereas in the human world the burden of representational anxieties is generally borne by women, who have to adjust appearance and behaviour to wider social and behavioural anxieties, in the doll world, males bear this burden of inadequacy. In recent years this issue has been masked when Ken and many other male dolls wore moulded Y-front underpants. They are permanently kept 'decent' and enterprising children cannot humiliate Ken and his peers by forcing them to go naked in public. Art historian Carol Ockman describes Ken's moulded briefs as 'an ingenious solution, for they manage to give the impression that there's something to hide without ever showing what that is' (Ockman 1999: 80).

Modern adult male dolls with full genitals are generally directed to a 'gay' market. They include Billy of 1997 and Bob of 1977, the latter often named by collectors as 'Gay Bob', affectionately and without disrespect. He was sold in a cardboard closet from which his owner could liberate him. Billy is famed amongst fashion dolls because, unlike his male or female compeers, his anatomy interferes with the stylish fit of his clothes (Houston-Montgomery 1999: 102), quite the opposite of euphemised Ken, but often equally the target of mocking comment. Many recent Barbie dolls have floral patterns stamped on their plastic hips and crotch to demonstrate that they are permanently dressed in briefs. Some wear spray-painted pants or bikinis to keep them permanently covered. These substitutions look more surreal than modest. The shape of the hip joints means that the section with moulded floral patterns does not look like any undergarment currently worn by women. This emphasises the unrealness of the jointing and form of the Barbie body. For costing production, permanently moulded-on underwear is cheaper than providing Barbie or Ken with sewn fabric knickers. Bourgeois capitalism wins out over bourgeois morality. Mostly, the more expensive Barbie dolls for adult collectors wear full underwear. Often their lingerie is carefully coordinated with the doll's overall persona. Empress Elisabeth of Austria from 1996 wears long white Victorian bloomers and the second Christian Dior Barbie from 1996, in her 1947 dress, wears stylish black briefs and suspenders.

Fashion dolls not only deliver a supposedly 'inappropriate' sexuality to young girls, as well as being sexual/sexualised performers themselves, in the mind of the prudent and puritanical the fashion doll encourages 'foolish' girls and women to buy, buy, buy: each new dress, each new edition, to be a stooge, a running dog of capitalism. Barbie is regarded as an education in consumerism and Mattel is believed to exemplify the hegemonical strategies of a malign capitalism (Rand 1995: 2–9, 26–29, 144–8; Rogers 1999: 71–75, 86–91, 95; Varney 2002: 41–43). The modern dolls derived from the German character doll – the living, 'new born' babies and the 'natural' children of modern German dollmakers such as Annette Himstedt and Hildegarde Günzel – are frequently seen as more appropriate items to place in the hands of children. It is perhaps one of fashion's slyest and most *unheimlich* stratagems that those who abhor 'fashion' and despise the fashion doll's 'inappropriate' colonisation of an 'innocent' childhood jump out of Barbie's capitalist frying pan into the *völkisch* fire of the German 'character' doll. The latter's studied realism and naturalism assert the purity of humanity and an emotionally direct communication: a utopian desire for a life that is simple, frugal, diligent and adorned by the dignity of service and the beauty of nature. Fashion's mirrorball ironically illuminates its enemies' strange left-right confluence.

This history informs the 'Barbie is cheap/unnatural' discourse. The debates about the physical form of the psychologically healthy doll led to the semi-official disappearance of dolls with adult identities and personae. Adult female dolls, for centuries a doll trade staple, did not find favour with early-twentieth-century professional discourses on doll design. 'A doll representing a woman, dressed up like an adult, such as formerly were by far in the majority, cannot awaken maternal feelings in the little girl, for she can not easily descry her child in the shape of a lady of fashion' (von Boehn 1966: 175). An article credited by present-day German author Sabine Reinelt to an early-twentieth-century German journal the *Toys, Jewellery and Sports Article* review of 1910 stated that 'a doll should not be a lady, not a lace covered being in a delicate silk dress, it should represent a child . . . that can awaken an illusion in the heart of the little mother: this is your child . . . The impression that the usual doll makes lies purely in their external appearance' (Reinelt 1993: 92–93). Defining the 'elegant fashion doll' as 'an unnatural object' (von Boehn 1966: 177) suggests that the language of criticism directed at Barbie, especially in relation to her wardrobe and her role as 'fashion' doll, has a much longer historical presence. Such prehistories may prompt questions as to what is actually being objected to in modern fashion dolls. Questions could also be raised as to what type of doll is being nominated as substitute for the despised fashion doll. Mainstream academic literature is problematised. An example is Humphrey McQueen's essay on Barbie, in which he suggests that 'girls did not mother her but admired her' (1998: 127) is problematised. Likewise in the 1990s Miriam Formanek-Brunell upholds the turn-of-the-century idea that 'dolls resembling fashionable ladies . . . were intended for neither soothing nor cuddling' (1993: 13).

Adult-styled dolls disappeared so rapidly from public memory that both Barbie's physiology and her deep involvement with fashion are routinely defined as aberrant. The preceding paragraphs indicate, however, that the norm is by no means as neutral or benign as is generally assumed. Like the white wedding, the intervention of authorities to maintain the endangered foetus in the aberrant female body, and other traditions that supposedly indicate the 'stability' of the family, the idea that the appropriate image for the doll is a baby to be mothered is relatively new and dates from the beginnings of the twentieth century. It is too easy to assume, given the dearth of other evidence, that Barbie brought sex – adult and modern – into the doll universe of the 1950s, 'a world of baby dolls and little girl dolls' (McDonough 1999: 13), as a microscopic version of the modernist revolution, but in fact the postwar dollworld was already far more knowing and intertextually alert than has been assumed. Moreover whatever directives were imposed by the product, the general public resisted the social engineering that 'experts' sought to promulgate through 'correct' dolls. Despite the relative paucity of dolls designed as adults, many families and owners who wanted an adult-personaed doll simply dressed dolls, characterised by their makers as infants or children, in adult clothes. This adult dressing looks particularly strange against the childlike faces and features when specialised garments such as nuns' habits or soldiers' uniforms are intended to be represented. Likewise those responsible for the profusion of home-dressed Queen Elizabeth II portrait dolls in gala evening dress during the 1950s and 1960s had no alternative than to employ dolls with childlike facial modelling, despite the fact that the dolls were often intended to portray high-formal garments such as the coronation vestments or the robes of state.

La Renaissance de la Poupée Française

The extent of French dollmaking beyond the Société Française de Fabrications de Bébés et Jouets in the period 1900–1914 is hard to estimate. Gesland and Steiner survived as individual companies, as did mechanical-toy manufacturers such as Leopold Lambert and Roullet et Decamps, the latter made many walking dolls. The Huret moulds began to be used again in the early 1900s by Elisa Prevost who engaged in small-scale studio manufacture of bisque dolls. Damerval also possibly manufactured bisque heads before the First World War. The artist and cartoonist François Poulbot was designing and exhibiting cloth dolls by 1908. Wax dolls in modern and historic fashions were made well before the First World War, during the first decade of the twentieth century, by two sisters under their married names of Lafitte and Desirat (Coleman et al. 1986: 686). On her husband's side Madame Lafitte was the sister-in-law of the founder of the well-known Parisian fashion journal *Femina*. In 1902 a prize was offered to artists to design the perfect French doll with submissions by École des Beaux Arts luminaries such as Fremiet, Detaille and Gérôme, but no commercially viable models emerged (von Boehn 1966: 186). French dolls kept their reputation as fashion ambassadors throughout the early-twentieth century. 'Doll dressmaking in Paris is a genuine science for the Parisian article, like her human counterpart of that city, takes the fashions with her everywhere. All her dainty clothing are [sic] perfect copies of the apparel of the women who are seen on the Boulevards of the French capital' (*Toys and Novelties*, 1913; qtd Coleman et al. 1986: 281).

Some accounts suggest that few dolls were made in France between 1900 and 1914 and many companies were dependent upon parts imported from Germany (*Toys and Novelties*, date unknown, and Leo Claretie, 1918; both qtd Coleman et al. 1986: 434). However such accounts may also be influenced by the sense of heightened crisis and hysteria typical of the war years. In May 1915 Georges d'Avenel in the *Revue des Deux Mondes* claimed that over the past fifteen years the SFBJ had upgraded the capacity of the Jumeau kilns approximately sixfold and could fire 30,000 dolls' heads at a time (d'Avenel 1915: 346); this suggests that the SFBJ was certainly producing dolls' heads in France at that period. Pierre Calmette wrote a 1924 history of toys (qtd Coleman et al. 1986: 768) which stated that the SFBJ only returned to French manufactured heads during the war and continued into the 1920s. The SFBJ was always commended for its deeply serious approach to fashion. In c.1900 one Laura S. Farlow said that the SFBJ 'employs thousands of hands and in certain cases takes as much trouble over frocks and hats as Worth or Paquin do in the case of real live grown ups'. '[D]ressmaking for smart dolls is a mightily elaborate business to which Paris devotes much of her marvellous art' (qtd Coleman et al. 1986: 767). It was suggested that in the 1920s the workrooms of the SFBJ had as good facilities and equipment as companies making clothes for adults (Coleman et al. 1970: 83) and that the SFBJ was proactive in gauging fashion trends (1970: 586). From the evidence of surviving dolls in original clothes, the SFBJ was one of the few doll companies in any country to actively respond to the *garçonne* style in 1920s fashion, and dress dolls in shift dresses and cloche hats, often in brightly coloured real silks for expensive models and artificial rayons for the cheaper ones.

After 1914, ceramic studios including Damerval, Lanternier and J. Verlinge produced dolls for the French domestic market. These dolls never matched the quality of earlier French dolls, although some seem to have been copied or cast from Jumeau dolls (Jaeger 2000: 76–7). Incised on these later French dolls are names such as Chéri, La Favourite, Caprice, Petite Française, ToTo, and the different moulds evoke popular attitudes towards women in early-twentieth-century France as well as current politics. The doll bearing the name Lorraine speaks of the bitterly mourned lost province and indicates that these dolls have nationalist references. Another model is incised with the name Liane, perhaps representing the French courtesan Liane de Pougy, who was known to the public as the 'Nation's Lianon'. There was much public affection for Liane as she was a French woman, whereas her rivals Caroline 'La Belle' Otéro, Lina Cavallini and

Cléo de Mérode were Spanish, Italian and Belgian respectively (de Pougy 1977: 13).

Cutting off supplies of dolls from Germany, the key international source of dolls in 1914 caused a crisis that was solved by an intense new wave of dollmaking and experimentation. The United States and Britain, both of which may have made a small amount of bisque dolls before the war,[2] stepped up production by several firms, such as the British Goss factory, famed for its heraldic souvenir china. Italy, Belgium, Spain, Russia, as well as areas still gazetted in Austria pre-1914 and later in the Czech Republic, also manufactured dolls' heads in various kinds of ceramic from porcelain to stoneware. Japan rapidly moved in to supply the United States market. In a few years the doll industry had become as lucrative to the Japanese economy as it had been to the German and the French economies. There was a serious downturn when, by the early 1920s, the North Americans renewed their close contacts with the German doll industry and stopped buying Japanese product. However in some markets, such as Australia, the Japanese celluloid baby doll remained a staple right through the interwar years. Japan produced millions of cheap novelty bisque dolls throughout the 1920s and 1930s. These little figurines were not only used as children's toys but often given away as party favours, table decorations and corsages at adult dances and functions in the interwar years.

During the 1914–18 war there was a renewed interest in rag dolls due to war-time shortages. Rag dolls became a popular substitute for ceramic dolls, even though the make-do-and-mend ethos was not so formally emphasised in the First World War as in the second. The necessities of wartime shortages coincided with cultural discussion about the role of art, design and handcraft in doll and toy production. Ironically in view of the wartime context such issues were inspired by the German doll reform movement and the Wiener Werkstätte's exploration of children's toys, especially folkcrafts and handwork in wood, cloth and paper. The avant-garde aspect of this Central European scrutiny of toys was concerned with the elaboration and over-refinement of materials, designs and substances used in industrially produced toys. The war accelerated an existing impetus towards exploring 'humble', handworked toys and the role of good design in children's lives.

A number of different cloth dolls from the First World War period can be identified. In France small dolls made from hanks of wool, silk or cotton thread tied in bundles were very popular as good luck charms for civilians and soldiers alike in dangerous situations. Such dolls were carried in the pocket or worn around the neck like a scapular (Coleman et al. 1986: 863). As a young woman, the famous North American doll industry matriarch, 'Madame' Beatrice Alexander began making cloth dolls in New York to fill the gap in the market left by the lack of German bisque dolls. The Paderewski rag dolls were fundraisers for Polish refugees. They were promoted by Madame Paderewski, wife of the famous pianist and statesman. Madame Lazarski employed war widows and wives of soldiers serving at the front to sew rag dolls for her *Ateliers Artistiques* in Paris. Marie Vassilief made modern-styled rag dolls in Russia, and by the First World War was running a 'modern art' school in Paris. Vassilief knew various revolutionary exiles (she had, it was claimed in the press, even served a jail term for revolutionary activities), and commenced dollmaking again in Paris after the outbreak of the war. A number of these French studios and makers were closely associated, and worked together in production or marketing, or looked covertly or overtly to each other's production for inspiration and new directions. Some primary accounts of these dolls are confused and make vast-ambit claims for each or various of these studios. The extremity and exaggeration of these accounts are influenced by the heady and emotionally intense experiences of public life during war when the success of the dolls was often tied up with fundraising for worthy causes or assisting those suffering or displaced due to the war. An interesting example of such journalism was reprinted by the Coleman family from the *Brooklyn Eagle*, although no date is given. It indicates how couture studios turned to dollmaking to keep hands employed:

> During World War One[3] a new type of cloth doll was created by Mme Vassilief which inspired the Madame Paderewski dolls. Copies of the Vassilief dolls were made by the first hands in the workrooms of famous French dressmakers. But the copies had no real artistic merit when compared with the original Vassilief dolls. (qtd Coleman et al. 1986: 1171)

Concurrently British toy companies printed rag dolls onto calico, including soldiers and little girls. These dolls were printed in two or more parts on flat cloth to be cut out and sewn together to make a soft three-dimensional toy. Such printed rag dolls had been an American advertising fad since the late-nineteenth century, but they acquired renewed currency in First World War Britain. Like the paper dolls so popular in the Second World War, printed rag dolls were vivid, appealing, with minimum use of materials. Detail and personality were conveyed through graphic printing rather than time and labour consuming moulding or production of second-ary accessories such as shoes, clothes, wigs, eyes, stringing elastic, all of which would take up both resources and person power that could have been directed to the war effort. Wartime advertisements in Australian women's journals advertised these printed dolls. Mail order houses sent them out as flat sheets for mothers to sew, stuff and finish. Large-sized dolls could be effectively dressed in cast-off children's clothes, so the wholesaler advised (Fainges 1993: 14). Sharing cast-off clothes with the doll indicated responsible wartime thrift and management of pre-existing resources. Ironically one of these British wartime printed rag dolls was drawn carrying a naturalistic bear doll, perhaps intended to reference the 'Russian bear', the great ally, but it looked more like the bear featured on the Berlin coat of arms, thus making quite the opposite statement about wartime loyalties than the designer perhaps intended. These wartime printed dolls received a new lease of life when some were reproduced during the 1970s as souvenirs of the Victoria and Albert Museum.

In France, wartime conditions, the reduced supply of German dolls, the intensive hyperpatriotism of a country at war, and the cumulative effects of decades of the statutory hostility of the Third Republic to Germany begot a movement called *La Renaissance de la Poupée Française*. Artistic doll exhibitions for wartime charities were frequently held in Paris, and sometimes exported to support the war effort and send the Allies a timely reminder of *La Gloire de France*. Jeanne Doin saw the appearance of new dolls as a natural result of the war, a sort of hyper-essentialism of gender difference begotten by wartime conditions: 'Thus runs the world. Men take up arms and little girls dolls.' Dolls were as necessary as armaments (Doin 1916: 433). The revival in French dollmaking was also partly a response to both the English Arts and Crafts movement and the early-twentieth-century German Doll reform movement. As in Germany, Austria and the United States, the French movement towards scrutinising the aesthetic elements of dolls related to the general interest in raising the standard of design in consumer goods. This theorised dollmaking could be linked to the avant-garde gestures in France that intensified in the years prior to the First World War. The orientalist fervour begotten by the colour palettes, movement and radical design of the Diaghilev ballet, as well as the interest in 'reforming' fashion spoken most showily by Paul Poiret and more subtly by Fortuny, Paquin and Madeleine Vionnet, then in the very early stages of her career, also provided a context in which dolls could be re-evaluated. Jeanne Doin even suggested that the dolls of Madame Ciechanowska 'evoked distant memories of [Diaghilev's] *Schéhérazade*' (Doin 1916: 448).

As well as the patriotic need to create a 'French' doll independent from German influence, this modernist issue of the simplification of form and design in toys, the removal of superfluous elements of decoration, the use of abstraction and synthesis to capture the expressive essence of a character or form is constantly reiterated when discussing the 'new' French dolls of the war era and their dressing. Jeanne Doin in the *Gazette des Beaux Arts* praises Madame Pierre Goujon who designed new costumes to remake 'ordinary dolls' through their fashions. Goujon rejected 'pink and blue satin' doll dresses now obsolete with their 'falballas, feathers, bows, laces, fake *guipure* of the "*modèle riche*" . . . It is too convenient to always reproduce the same ideas. Less expensive fabrics, more diverse styling and *voilà* the wardrobe of the rejuvenated doll' (Doin 1916: 442). Doin also suggested that the creators of the new dolls were 'animated' by a sense of 'simplification' in the forms and the limbs of the dolls (1916: 438). The mimetic poupée and bébé with their luxury dresses were increasingly out of touch with a new aesthetic of the expressive avant-garde rag doll. Over the winter of 1916/1917 the Paris-based Musée des Arts Décoratifs held an exhibition in the Pavilion de Marsan at the Louvre of *Images et Jouets, Artistiques et Modernes* which featured many of these radical wartime rag dolls and redesigned dolls. The exhibition clearly defined these wartime dolls as *moderne*. This was an official acknowledgement of the importance of these new-styled dolls and toys to the French spirit and self-image during the war.

Rather than following the realist psychological veracity of German dolls, the French asserted French style and specialised handwork and hand-finishing over the naturalism and anti-fashion gestures of the middle European doll reform. Due to exigencies of war these new French dolls were produced in limited, studio-sized production runs, rather than industrial volume. High-quality dollmaking became neither a frivolous gesture nor an indication of women's feebleness and doll-like identity, but was a serious representation of the French nation, just as Emile-Louis Jumeau had claimed on behalf of his dolls three decades earlier. When dolls took centre stage in patriotic demonstrations, renowned couturiers added prestige to these important performances of the French spirit. Dolls kept skilled hands on the payroll of Haute Couture ateliers during the war. Lack of money, restricted low-key social events and increasing numbers of widows in high society, who withdrew from social life and wore dress severely limited by social convention, all reduced the customer base of couture houses. Loyal customers were ordering less, as they had fewer opportunities to display new dresses.

As with the Théâtre de la Mode in 1945, if fabrics were in short supply, and prices were at a premium for goods of decent quality, presenting couture garments in a fraction of adult size became a feasible solution to erratic and limited supply chains and prohibitive pricing. During both World Wars the doll became a prototype for French couture, showing what could be envisaged full-sized when conditions returned to normal. This confluence of patriotism, propaganda and French couture appears in an exhibition of bisque dolls dressed by the Callot Sisters as part of a display of French dolls held by the American Art Alliance in New York in 1917 (D.S. and E.J. Coleman 1989: 95). The *Revue des Deux Mondes* in May 1915 explicitly stated that 'last autumn', 1914, saw the 'rebirth' of 'coquettishly dressed lady dolls', under the patronage of society ladies, and made by the *'petits mains'* of the couture houses, with heads designed by major sculptors. In peacetime both the sculptors and the seamstresses making these dolls had been engaged in the expected work of their *métiers*. Now dollmaking was proving a practical outlet for their talents. The dolls were made and dressed from scraps lying around ateliers and shops (d'Avenel 1915: 351). Jeanne Doin claimed that during the war the fashion doll was being revived for her original purpose of promoting French fashions 'because voyages are risky and salesmen are rare' (1916: 449).

An example of these new dolls were the Huret-Prevost dolls. Elisa Prevost, a relatively young woman, with a 'feel' for the avant-garde, bought the doll moulds and business name of Adelaide Huret before the war. She had started limited production and her artistic dolls were well placed to be taken up by *La Renaissance de la Poupée Française*. A number of the Huret-Prevost dolls survive in couture costumes by Jeanne Lanvin in the collection of the Musée des Arts Decoratifs, Paris. These dolls have had relatively little publicity down the years. François Theimer illustrates some of these dolls, suggesting that they date from around the end of the First World War (Theimer 1999: 58–9). The detailing on the dolls is superb, especially the choice of fabrics, which include the metallic laces so popular at this period, intricate cornelli machine embroidery (a standard in French embellishment of dresses and underwear through to the Second World War) and a dress cut from exotic Egyptian asyut silver-embroidered cloth. The millinery is particularly elaborate on such a small scale. Lanvin also dressed dolls with glazed china heads made during the war at the National Manufactory at Sèvres. One was illustrated in Antonia Fraser's book on dolls (1964: 44), but generally Lanvin's Sèvres dolls have been invisible in the English language fashion press. The doll illustrated by Fraser has a dress that appears nostalgic at first glance, but has radical detailing such as an asymmetrically draped skirt, no actual pannier or crinoline support and an overall chinoiserie feel. Large-scale oriental-style fringing decorates the skirt and the diagonal bodice closure is a simplified interpretation of Chinese court costume. The Colemans claim that these Lanvin dolls were given to the Louvre by Margaine-Lacroix (1986: 690).

Lanvin's Huret dolls are dressed in current fashions. Theimer (1999: 58) picks up on the characterisation of the dolls made by Prevost and, in some cases, modelled by her, and regards them as expressing a 'modern' spirit in their 'austere, androgynous' personae. Theimer links them to the legendary man-woman of the 1830s, George Sand, but the dolls resemble the British patroness of the avant-garde Ottoline Morel, who was well known in *Ballets Russes* circles. The dolls evoke the dramatic, mannerist characterisation of women seen in the art of Romaine Brooks. Coincidentally one of Sand's granddaughters, Madame Lauth-Sand, made artistic rag dolls during the war in France (Coleman et al. 1986: 693). Elisa Prevost's dolls are distinctly women of the early-twentieth century, whereas the dolls by Adelaide Huret were quintessential characterisations of the women of her era: the Second Empire. As Theimer notes '[t]wo women separated by half a century made dolls that were in perfect harmony with their times' (1999: 59). Elisa Prevost and Jeanne Lanvin were friends (Theimer 1999: 58) thus facilitating the link between the dolls and the couturière. Jeanne Lanvin had other links to the French doll industry. She knew the family who ran *La Semaine de Suzette*, and assisted in the design of some of the models for the magazine's premium doll, Bleuette, sold through the publisher's Parisian offices. These ready-made clothes followed in the popularity of the paper patterns offered in the magazine (Theimer 1993b: 5, 7). Lanvin is even believed to have provided offcuts from her atelier for these dresses (Billyboy 2003).

The most famous dolls from the First World War were designed by Albert Marque and dressed by Jeanne Margaine-Lacroix. These dolls are legendary amongst collectors, and are regarded as the rarest and most expensive of all historic dolls. For Mildred Seeley, the memorable element of the Marque dolls was not that they were extremely rare and desirable, but instead their identity as sculptures, rather than industrial production. The Marque dolls' singular, self-contained nature was paramount for Seeley. Their style and manner of modelling had relatively little relation to known formats of mainstream factories and she hypothesised that the Marque dolls were beyond the range and vision of 'an ordinary dollmaker' (Seeley 1992: 6–8, 54).

Research by Mildred Seeley (1993: 54–7) and François Theimer (Anon 1998: 29) has identified the careers of those responsible for the production of the Marque dolls. The dolls can be firmly dated to the First World War, but the exact circumstances of how they were produced, and how a fine art sculptor and Paris' leading corsetière came to collaborate on a doll still remains obscure. The production of a doll by professional artists beyond the doll trade again testifies to the iconic status that dolls held for the French during the First World War. Margaine-Lacroix was an establishment of the first rank in Parisian couture, although not widely discussed in histories of fashion. Mother and daughter Margaine-Lacroix won the gold medal at the 1889 Paris exhibition for corsetry and the grand prix at the 1900 exhibition. At the beginning of the First World War the younger Margaine-Lacroix was still one of the most prominent of names in corsetry in Paris, having registered a number of trademarks and patents for foundation garments during the previous two decades.

Albert Marque was a well-known and respected sculptor at the turn of the century, described by a French critic as the 'friend of small children' (Seeley 1992: 54), a specialist in child subjects. This focus upon child subjects would have made Marque extremely popular in early-twentieth-century France in the wake of concerns about repopulation and stabilising the birth rate that became a widespread obsession following the Franco-Prussian War. When showing alongside radical painters, Marque was described by a reviewer as '*Donatello au milieu des fauves*' – Donatello amongst the wild beasts – at the Salon d'Automne of 1905 (Anon 1998: 28). This critical comment on Marque may have begotten the now-accepted name of the Fauves art movement. Artworks by Marque located by doll collectors have affinities with the radical sculptures of Mailloil and Bourdelle, who presented an earthy primitivism and broader stylisation of the classical style in the early-twentieth century. Instead of the mimetic detail of Beaux Arts classicism. Marque's particular stylistic signature was a mannerist, expressionist exaggeration of facial features into a series of triangulated points.

This individualistic, arbitrary, almost cubist treatment of form appears in the doll, although somewhat smoothed out by the bisque. The body is unlike those of other contemporary dolls, more abstracted and dramatic in comparison to ordinary dolls. The maker's name is unknown. Possibly the Albert Marque dolls were made in a ceramics studio that did not usually make dolls. Later writers generally believe that the dolls were made as artistic display pieces and not intended for play. An emotive essay captures the histrionic emotions behind the endeavour of dollmakers to expunge the German doll from public consciousness:

> the dolls were never intended as play objects, but rather to appeal to the adult worshipper of 'all things French'. Here, in the middle of war with Germany, was the ultimate snub of [sic] German dolls. A truly French doll singular, unlike any other in doll history either in the model of the head or the body, bearing the name of an illustrious French artist, sold in a medal winning Parisian boutique, costumed to represent royalty of regions of France. (Anon 1998: 29)

Dolls in original dress bear the label of Margaine-Lacroix. The majority of dolls currently known wear French provincial costumes. Some are dressed as males. One set of dolls that Margaine-Lacroix sold to the Carnegie Museum in April 1916, before the United States entered the First World War, was dressed as various historic French queens: Queen Isabel, Queen Marie, Queen Marie-Antoinette, Empress Josephine and Empress Eugénie. Other dolls are dressed in ultra-fashionable children's clothes, such as the girl in a flaring wartime crinoline, in bright blue/cerise tartan, which passed through Sotheby's in 1998 (Brittaine 2001: 57). Margaine-Lacroix sold a wide range of ceremonially dressed dolls during the war. The Carnegie Museum bought no less than thirty-five SFBJ dolls from her. Again these more ordinary dolls were dressed as notable French men and women in history.

Even everyday dolls wore patriotic clothes. The department store Printemps' 1918 catalogue included dolls dressed as girls from Alsace, nurses and Allied soldiers, the soldiers were 'carefully dressed'. An especially fine doll was named '*la Petite Americaine*' (qtd Coleman et al. 1986: 960–61). French postcards for children published during the war show a similar range of dolls with wartime personalities. Girl dolls were dressed as *Alsaciennes* and Red Cross nurses. Boy dolls were dressed in military uniforms of the Allies including kilted Scotsmen. One postcard (see Figure 5.1) showed two bisque dolls in crêpe-paper costumes, the larger, a girl in Alsatian ethnic costume, cold-shoulders a smaller doll dressed as a German infantryman. 'Go away Prussian! I don't want to play with you' says the patriotic French doll. Mildred Seeley illustrates a number of SFBJ dolls as indication of different moulds produced by the company, but neglects to mention their outstanding wartime costumes (Seeley 1992: 84). They are dressed as mem-

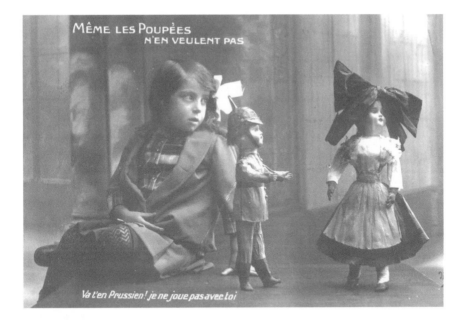

Figure 5.1 *Meme les Poupées n'en veulent pas: va t'en Prussien! je ne joue avec toi.* Postcard by JM, Paris c.1914–1918.

bers of the Allied armies, including a very elaborate Serbian. The French, Italian and Serbian dolls are officers, with swords and medals, but the British doll is a simple Tommy Atkins, suggesting that the SFBJ may have sold dolls dressed as both officers and privates.

The Princesses' Dolls

Patriotism and conditions of extremity twice again begot a singular revival of the French fashion doll. A distinct lineage runs from the dolls of the First World War to the couturier Bébés Jumeaus presented by the French government to the English princesses in 1938 as the French–British alliance was cemented just on the eve of the Second World War, through to the celebrated assertion of couture's survival after the war in the miniature-format couture display Le Théâtre de la Mode. The 'Princesses' Dolls' prefigured the Théâtre de la Mode in both the exclusive names of the contributing designers and the symbolic national mission. France's traumatic, but finally triumphant, survival of the Second World War was framed by the appearance of singular, beautiful Haute Couture dolls. In turn the Théâtre de la Mode, when it toured the United States, inspired American dollmaker Effanbee to commission Elsa Schiaparelli to design doll clothes and Madame Alexander to offer a fashionable lady, Cissy, as a regular line in her doll range. The success of Alexander's Cissy led to the release of Barbie. Billyboy's 1985 Mattel-endorsed collection of Barbies wearing international designer clothing was named Le Nouveau Théâtre de la Mode, translated as the New Theatre of Fashion in its North American tour and in subsequent English-language publications. Therefore the cross-reference, the homage in this 1980s exhibition of doll-sized high fashion, was explicit. This 'Nouveau' exhibition celebrated the achievements of couture in the mid-1980s, even if it did not share the extreme political and existential import-ance of the original, phoenix-like reappearance of French fashion in the inter-national marketplace as performed by the 1945 collection of miniature garments. Le Nouveau Théâtre codified adult and fashion history responses to Barbie, bringing a covert movement amongst isolated individuals out of the closet of personal obsession into the full, public light of theoretical and cultural credibility. Finally, when restored to the format of its 1946 North American tour and shown again, the dolls, scene settings and tableaux of the Théâtre, in its 1990 Metropolitan Museum installation, demonstrated to Mel Odom how appealing classic postwar fashion could be in miniature size (Anon 2001: 8; Sarasohn-Kahn 2001b). Odom's realisation directly led to the production of his Gene doll, who broke Barbie's monopoly on doll sales. In 2001 dollmaker Robert Tonner presented his own licensed versions of dresses from the Théâtre de la Mode. All these significant developments in dolls emerged from the United States, but were signposted by the Théâtre de la Mode.

The notable change from the nineteenth to the twentieth century is that, whereas the fashionable French doll was the norm for many decades in the nineteenth century, she only appeared at moments of extremity in the first half of the next century. The fashion doll reappeared when French sovereignty and identity were under threat during the First World War, in the late-1930s when Hitler's trajectory of confrontation with countries adjoining the German borders was unmistakable, or when order must be drawn from chaos and the pieces must be picked up again. These patriotic displays of dolls indicate how the supposedly trivial, feminine and frivolous world of dolls and fashion is symbolically intertwined with the public agora.

The first of these singular reappearances of the French fashion doll was the 1938 SFBJ gift to the two British Princesses. The moral and political sentiments behind these dolls are for some commentators still current, as demonstrated by the Royal Insight website. Its anonymous author emphasised the serious issues that shadowed the July 1938 state visit to France by King George VI and Queen Elizabeth. It 'was intended to consolidate the alliance of the democracies against the fascist threat; the Second World War was to break out just over a year later' (Royal Insight 2001). At the time of this state visit, the wife of the President of France developed the idea (Theimer 1998: 3) that an appropriate gift for the two royal princesses would be two dolls perfectly dressed and accessorised by the most desirable names in French couture. These dolls were produced as Bébé Jumeaus, therefore fulfilling the ideals of Emile-Louis Jumeau who in the 1880s and 1890s had considered his bébés to be the *Jouet National* as the Bébé Jumeau boxlids proclaimed. The national toy herself was a footsoldier for France ever ready to combat the evil and cheap German dolls. A new face mould was designed with the slender and svelte lines of 1930s beauty. The royal Bébé Jumeaus' wardrobe includes both children's and adults' clothes and implies simultaneously adult and child lifestyles. They are supplied with cots and prams, but also wear sensuous adult lingerie and have elaborate gowns for evening functions and garden parties, which suggests that they were society ladies. The postcards of the dolls issued to raise money for charity show them sometimes as children and sometimes as vampish young women, living an independent life. Their original names were France and Marianne but they were known colloquially as Elizabeth and Margaret. As well as dresses, which include models from 1938 collections, they have a legendary collection of women's accessories: fans painted by Marie Laurencin, jewellery by Cartier, luggage and handbags by Hermès and Vuitton, perfume by Lancôme and Guerlain. Perhaps the most frivolous and remarkable of their garments are their fur coats, including an ocelot three-quarter-length coat. There are also some extra items of furniture and accessories, including a small Citroën car and porcelain tea services. All the materials and craft skills were the best that the whole range of French luxury industries could offer.

The new mould designed for the Princesses' gift was reproduced commercially by the SFBJ in two sizes. Some of the surviving dolls are dressed by the company's workrooms in effervescent, filmy adult evening and garden party frocks, which reference the directions of the couture garments by such designers as Patou, Maggy Rouff and Jeanne Lanvin in the original gift. These 1938 Jumeaus are perhaps the most evocative and beautiful dolls produced during the 1930s, matched only by the very different sassy and sexy paper doll ladies being produced in the United States. These elegant bisque ladies are neither cute nor infantile and display more consistent workmanship than many regular SFBJ dolls. By their exceptional quality, the 1938 Jumeau/SFBJ dolls indicate how far dollmaking had been driven out of the world of contemporary art and design by psychologists and child theorists. When seen in context with the dolls of mid- to late-nineteenth-century France and the explosion of 'designer' dolls from the 1980s onwards, the 1938 Jumeau/SFBJ dolls serve to indicate how much style and elegance in miniature has been lost by the de facto severing of dollmaking from mainstream fashion culture in the interwar era. Ironically the 1938 dolls drew their focus and strength, as did the 1945 mannequin/dolls of the Théâtre de la Mode, from the nearly forgotten tradition of high-quality dollmaking in nineteenth-century France and the intense, patriotic sentiments around the conscious revival of dollmaking during the First World War.

On the eve of the war these superlative dolls also provided an entrée for couture into public consciousness. Rather than being used as toys by the two royal daughters (Elizabeth hardly being of a doll-playing age even by the standards of her generation), the dolls were assiduously employed as signs to proclaim the wonder of both the royal family and the mystique of Haute Couture. Their function as charity fundraisers and as political emblems of the struggle against fascism also neatly dissembles any cynical concern about the British royal family's hegemonic concentration of assets and social power around themselves. The dolls were placed on display in London where the public marvelled at their beauty and saw at first hand iconic couture labels, perhaps for the first time in their lives, or at least more closely than on the stage or the screen. The dolls and their clothes also featured in newsreels of the era, thus further facilitating democratic knowledge of current French couture.

In 1940 French fashion was disseminated to an additional general audience by the celebrated album by Whitman, an American publisher of paper dolls, documenting the couturier wardrobes. The album was entitled *Cut Outs from the Dolls of the Royal Princesses of England Princess Elizabeth Princess Margaret Rose* and subtitled *Designs by the famous fashion designers of France Lucien LeLong, Jean Patou, Jeanette Blanchôt, Maggy Rouff, Alexandrine, Paquin, Agnes, Duvelleroy, Marcel Rochas, Le Mounier, Jeanne Lanvin, Jungman, Max, Troustellier, Weil.* Thus the paper doll set became a means of circulating the names of well-known designers to an audience that would never be able to buy the originals. The fact that the designers were described as 'famous' indicates the importance of these designers by reputation alone to women and buyers of clothes, even if actual garments are not being bought or sold. These paper dolls of the *Dolls of the Royal Princesses of England* underpin the importance of the interchange between Haute Couture and dolls represented by the French government's gift to the Princesses.

As with the original dolls made for the Princesses, the image of the paper doll collection is dysphasic. The basic paper dolls that model the dresses are childlike in form and lingerie. They wear modest white panties and singlets and have flat chests, no bras and relatively straight contours on their torsos. Likewise the dolls' white ankle socks and flat shoes denote their child identity. However the dresses in the booklet are floor-length adult-style gowns, evening dresses, formal dresses and dresses for garden parties (following the printed descriptions), modified by the straight waistlines of the provided cardboard dolls (see Figure 5.2). The accessories – fur coats, long gloves and fans – are those of adult women. The dresses are rendered in three-colour printing from wash drawings, more prosaic and mimetic than the accepted style of fashion illustration of the period. Due to the immature forms of the dolls, everything perhaps lacks an essential final chic, but the set is of great historic importance in tracking popular-culture consciousness of couture, prior to the New Look capturing the attention of a wide class base.

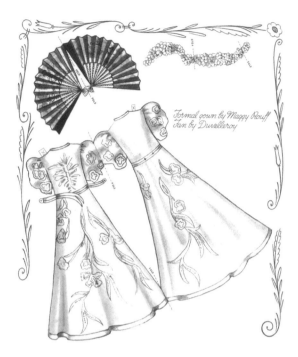

Figure 5.2 Formal gown by Maggy Rouff, fan by Duvelleroy from *Cut Outs from the Dolls of the Royal Princesses of England Princess Elizabeth Princess Margaret Rose*, Whitman USA, 1940.

Whitman's set of paper dolls of late-1930s French designers acts as a precedent to a more recent phenomenon: paper dolls based upon the work of major historic and contemporary couturiers. These dolls have been particularly popular amongst North American doll artists and collectors since the 1970s. Tom Tierney, the most prolific of modern paper-doll artists, has designed many sets of dolls accurately documenting the work of major couturiers from garments collected by museums, backed up through research in primary sources such as publicity photographs and advertising. Some of Tierney's doll albums are presented as a course in fashion history, and survey periods rather than designers. Other North American artists similarly research in museums and publications to produce adult collectors' paper dolls celebrating key designers and periods, again a refraction of high fashion's appeal to a populist audience.

The Théâtre de la Mode

The 'Princesses' dolls' have been eclipsed by a more famous, but closely related phenomenon, the Théâtre de la Mode: the defining event of postwar couture. The

Théâtre was a display of small doll-sized mannequins in painted and sculpted sets presented in the Pavilion de Marsan of the Louvre, in April 1945, even before VE Day. During the previous war the Pavilion had hosted patriotic doll exhibitions. The sculpting of the mannequins and design of the sets were by major French artists. Naturally the clothes and accessories were by named designers, as the project was expressly intended to demonstrate the survival of French couture and present the postwar collections, despite shortages. Over the past decade and a half the idea of the 'rebirth' of the Théâtre de la Mode has captured the attention of social and fashion historians. The phoenix-like reappearance of the actual dolls from 1945 (wearing the collections of Spring 1946) after their restoration and relaunch in the late 1980s has generated much copy. All accounts concur that the Chambre Syndicale de la Couture could not care less about the dolls being returned to France once they had fulfilled their original purpose of display and promotion, and virtually abandoned them (Anon 2002) after the expensive jewellery had been returned to France and accounted for at an official level. The fact that some of the dolls have always been on display for the past three decades at the Maryhill Museum (Anon 2002; Sarasohn-Kahn 2001b) is conveniently forgotten. The long chain of events between the disappearance of eighteenth-century fashion dolls as couriers and information sources and the Théâtre de la Mode has been effaced. Whilst the Princesses' dolls of 1938 provided a clear precedent for a cooperative public gathering of major couturiers and first-ranking accessory houses, they had left the country before the war, had been on public display to an English-speaking audience in Britain and Canada and had no clear place in the war-weary French public consciousness. Hence the Théâtre soon took on a magical dimension for its audience, thus pointing not only to a material and political victory, but also to a deliverance of the human spirit after the war. Over 100,000 people viewed the collection in Paris alone.

Houston-Montgomery's statement that 'the Théâtre de la Mode mannequins . . . gave credence to a new generation that dolls didn't have to resemble children (which up until the 1950s they usually did), but could actually fulfil the promise of adult sophistication . . .' (Houston-Montgomery 1999: 10) is arguable. As we have seen, throughout earlier periods the adult fashionable doll was the norm until s/he was defined as aberrant by medical and social theorists in the early-twentieth century. After the industrial revolution, the adult-styled Parisienne of c.1850–1880 enjoyed the offerings of a range of bespoke dressmakers and novelty houses, all made to her scale in styling and finish that matched adult couture. Moreover, and as discussed earlier, far from disappearing in the twentieth century, the fashionable doll had been revived at two earlier crisis points in French political life. The majority of subsequent commentators on the Théâtre de la Mode overlook its long and well-documented pedigree to a greater or lesser degree. The Lanvin house featured in all three major political reappearances of French fashion dolls. In the

First World War *Renaissance de la Poupée Française* Jeanne Lanvin dressed Huret and Sèvres dolls. France and Marianne wore Lanvin dresses as did the nameless figures of the Théâtre de la Mode. Certainly there is a disjunction between the consistent development of French couture from 1850 onwards and the disappearance of expensive French dolls of a similar quality in design and conception after 1900 as a marketplace staple, especially considering that both the luxury doll trade and the modern designer-driven couture had emerged at the same cultural moment in France.

The status of the figures in the Théâtre as 'dolls' is debatable, although the recent colonisation of the Théâtre by dollmakers and collectors is not. The anxieties about the figures' identity informs broader cultural discussion about fashion, women and dolls. The organisers strongly desired that the figures did not resemble 'dolls' or naturalistic figures. Perhaps this anxiety about representation signals the gulf between French high culture and dollmaking at that date, even though the Théâtre de la Mode is remembered amongst doll collectors as much as fashion historians. Perhaps this non-naturalism traces a self-consciously avant-garde interest in the abstract and non-representational, rather than the accessible and illustrative values of popular culture. The sculptor of the heads, Joan Rebull, a Catalan exile from fascism, asked that 'heads should not have makeup . . . they should be small sculptures' (Garfinkel 1991: 67). Here fine art/sculpture is pitted against fashion/appearances/female deception as symbolised by cosmetics. Whilst the Théâtre is nominally proclaimed as the survival of 'fashion' as a symbol to mark 'freedom' and a defiant French weathering of German occupation, at its heart is an ambiguity about fashion as a symbol of the feminine, the popular, the changeable and the surface neatly symbolised by 'makeup'.

The mannequins emphasised fine art values. The wire frameworks that the clothes were set upon had themselves a sculptural presence. Their graphic and scribbling freedom of outline recalls a number of esteemed artworks: Jean Cocteau's cleverly sparse caricatures, Picasso's classical drawings of the 1920s and the linear, antic outlines of Alexander Calder's early wire circus sculptures. 'Raw materials of any sort were difficult to come by, so wire was a "found" material (much like Pablo Picasso's "found" sculptures with bicycle seats-as-bull's horns)' (Sarasohn-Kahn 2001b). The format was a collaborative practice. Eliane Bonabel, a young illustrator who had additional experience in puppetry, devised the basic prototype of the wire mannequin. The heads were sculpted by Joan Rebull. Bonabel's concept was realised by Jean Saint Martin, a sculptor with a background in creating store mannequins for Siegel. The Siegel company gained fame in French art circles for developing an avant-garde, abstract image in shop mannequins that found a receptive audience in the 1920s. Siegel's acclaimed mannequins readily captured the attention of Surrealist artists (Charles-Roux 1991a: 33–4). Puppets and store mannequins were always more esteemed than dolls by the early- and mid-twentieth-century avant-garde as they were seen as creatures of greater agency and disjunctive powers than dolls, who are archetypally feminine and passive by implication.

Rilke wrote of a doll 'giving itself airs stolidly and mutely like some peasant Danaë knowing nothing but the ceaseless golden shower of our invention' (1994: 32). 'A poet could fall under the domination of a marionette, because the marionette has only imagination. A doll has none, and is exactly that much less of a thing as a marionette is more' (1994: 34). This dichotomy speaks of foundational tropes of the legend of modernist creativity, male/female, active/passive, agent/submissive, actor/acted upon, that explain the doll's general absence from mainstream cultural awareness throughout the twentieth century and her exile to the particular realm of her fans and collectors and their self-reflexive values. Thus in 1945 the Théâtre had to be carefully quarantined from the pollution that the doll as trivial, passive and female, threatened to bring to the project. Few took Rilke's next step of suggesting that the doll – like the *Mona Lisa* for Walter Pater – assumed a perverse power, as dominatrix, as femme fatale, in her stasis, her refusal to acknowledge or return the emotions invested in her by the sensitive male dreamer (1994: 34–9).

Surrealism and fashion marketing had a conjoined sensibility in the interwar and mid-century years (Caws 1997: 25–30) that informs the Théâtre. In the 1930s and onwards, dolls played only a minor part in this connection between fashion retailing and the avant-garde which famously extends through the surrealist fascination with the dummy to the interest of Walter Benjamin and Joseph Cornell in sites such as shops and arcades. Yet probing beneath the surface of this de facto intellectual/artistic scorn for dolls, primary sources around dolls suggest that they have a far greater affinity to these issues of display, commodification, replication and disjunction that had interested the avant-garde between the wars and had been taken up in turn by the fashion and fashion marketing industries in Europe and North America by the eve of the war.

Despite the positivist rejection of dolls as not cutting an appropriate level of cultural and intellectual ice, the Théâtre project itself did not seem quite resolved about the doll/mannequin/sculpture question. The 'life' of the dolls ebbs and flows through the early photographs of the project reproduced in the sumptuous album celebrating the restoration of Théâtre de la Mode (Charles-Roux 1991a: 33, 35). In some images they hang lifeless in their dozens from wires on hooks. Although dressed in spreading evening finery, they evoke the promiscuous loss of life in the not-quite-ended war and its new and horrifying forms of multiple death, so often recorded by cameras. Elsewhere the mannequins lie scattered in pieces across workroom tables evoking the horror film genre or Hans Bellmer's artworks. Like children, they are carried up staircases by human assistants. However, in some images they have life and emotions and thus interact with the people alongside them. Eliane Bonabel and one of her dolls stand side by side holding hands, both dressed in suits and wartime wedge shoes. The doll looks upwards at Eliane who inclines graciously to her companion. Perhaps it is an image to control and frame both woman artist and doll as problematic sisters of strangeness. The sorority and interchangeability of doll and woman are emphasised.

This effacing of the popular and the female, or this stated desire to efface the popular and the female partly reflects the surrealist 'problem of woman' and the intense ambiguity that the Surrealists read around women (Caws 1997: 35–9; Evans 1999: 3–32). The settings of the Théâtre demonstrate the elegant assimilation of surrealist tropes into fashion marketing, with such scenes as a carousel and an imaginary baroque garden. Jean Cocteau's set featured beauties in evening dresses posed in front of a crumbled wall. Suggesting either bomb damage or disjunctive slippages and fissures in the psyche; this surrealist tableau emphasised both women and fashion as strange and out of the ordinary. By associating fashion, beauty and the female with war damage it rendered them both as something to be feared (and there is a strong tradition of Germany being imaged as essentially feminine in the popular culture of both World Wars, for example as a priori treacherous, unreliable, inferior through such films as *Cabaret*, 1972, and *Zentropa*, 1991), but through this association of violence and unpredictability inferred by the woman-war analogy, women also became agents and begetters of the surrealist forces of disjunction and the unexpected, and the coming together of the seemingly contradictory, which is seen to perfection in Cocteau's juxtaposition of the pristine bell-shaped evening gowns and the crumbling masonry.

The strong moral imbrication of the Théâtre de la Mode with the serious events of 'world history' is frequently present in current discourse around the collection.

It was in a troubled climate of extremes that the Théâtre de la Mode came into being. A demonstration of determination against fortitude; the results of which probably surpassed all expected success. And even today, more than 50 years later, these small-size ambassadors of elegance still impress and move us. They possess a charisma which is timeless. Restrictions of the war, combined with the weather in Paris which was particularly cold during the winter months of 1944 with much snow on the ground, (an unusual occurrence for Paris) increased the hardships of the Parisians even more. But Paris had been liberated in August bringing expectations for better times and the possibility of a future reconstruction of industries. The country was still rampant as the daily struggle for the first necessities: food, heating, clothes went on. It was in this ambience of rigor and hope that the idea was born of proving that the French Haute Couture was not a thing of the past; that its vitality and supremacy were still intact and could still hold its place internationally. [punctuation sic] (Anon 2002b)

Like the Princesses' dolls this collection of fashionable ladies gains cultural credibility when they are enlisted in the great cause of the World War; this was an early indication of the public charitable display of such events as 'Style Aid'.

The Théâtre speaks of couture's travail during the Second World War. The lavish album published to document the restoration of the mannequins provides extended accounts of the complex negotiations of Lucien LeLong to ensure the survival of couture under the occupation. The rivalry between North American innovative couture, which came into its own during the war years, and French tradition is fully documented in the same album. Chanel, whose house was not in operation over the war years and who was regarded as a collaborator, was not included in the Théâtre; her absence provokes questions about the uncomfortable issues of French survival during the occupation. At the very least remembering the project brings forth thoughts of the privations of life at that era. 'Plagued by inadequate heating, electricity cuts, barely adequate food rations and often obliged to get to work on foot or on bicycles, the skilled tailors and seamstresses in the workrooms of the couturiers and milliners never the less threw themselves into the project with enthusiasm and fervour' (Garfinkel 1991: 68). '[T]here were shortages of every conceivable kind. The Chambre Syndicale had to obtain special government permits for the lumber and plywood used for the decors. Madame Scheikewitch (then Madame Robert Ricci) remembers finally locating a supply of plaster for the heads and delivering it to the workshop in her little gazigene runabout. The couturiers ransacked their stocks for scraps of fabric' (Garfinkel 1991: 71).

> How strange to recall all that in 1990; to evoke a past from which some of us will never truly recover, that past of inventions seized, art abolished and industry in ruins: a time of empty stomachs, of chapped lips, and shoes in holes; those days of submission and obedience to commands barked out by an invader whose voice was harsh and brutal. A bad memory. Better not dwell on it. Forty Five years ago already . . . (Charles-Roux 1991a: 28, 30)

Valerie Steele is a little less disingenuous. Part of the mission of the Théâtre was the necessity of 'emphas[ising] that Paris fashion had not been irrevocably contaminated by collaboration with the Nazis' and 'disarm[ing] foreign critics' (Steele 1997: 9). Considering that during the early-twentieth century both the French and the Germans read the fashion doll in nationalist terms, with the French seeing her as a sign of national prestige and the Germans seeing her as superficial and seeking to reform or improve on her, the mission of the mannequins of the Théâtre was historically well established.

The first collection involved 170 outfits from forty couturiers. It toured to a number of cities, including Vienna, with furs being added for the Stockholm showings. For the important American showing to win back customers from the extraordinarily creative wartime American couture there was a new set of spring 1946 outfits worn by an augmented rollcall of 237 mannequins. Jane Sarasohn-

Kahn notes that 'the tour was also very strategic in intent. Parisian fashion houses wanted desperately to win back their lost American clientele' (Sarasohn-Kahn 2001b). The surviving Théâtre is a substantial proportion of this second collection of mannequins and backdrops, restored in France in the 1980s. After lying in storage for some years it found an appropriate safe haven in the Maryhill Museum, an American art gallery, but dropped out of public knowledge.

Possibly the most important aspect of the Théâtre from a functional empirical fashion history perspective, beyond its intense metaphorical functions, is its documentation of houses that have not captured the attention of journalists, historians or curators in subsequent years. Its contextualised vision presents famous names alongside those known, when the collection was restored in the 1980s, only to ageing customers with long memories or professional specialists thoroughly familiar with the primary sources. A number of the labels included in the Théâtre were also considered important enough to dress France and Marianne before the war, however their importance has been written over by the titanic reputations of the iconic male designers of the postwar era. Some of these companies were headed by female designers such as Mad Carpentier and Maggy Rouff. The Théâtre assists in redressing the unbalanced theoretical and historical reticence around once highly regarded female designers and contributes to the still controversial debate about the female contribution to classic twentieth-century couture (Steele 1991: 9–17). Oblivion is not only a feminist issue: some lesser-known houses in the Théâtre were directed by male designers and their reputations have fallen as much as those of their female colleagues. Perhaps there is a generational issue with the postwar houses obscuring the achievements of those of the interwar and wartime years.

The Théâtre backs up a recent revisionist reading of fashion history, which suggests that the New Look of 1947 was more revolutionary in press coverage and propaganda than it was in design and structure (McDowell 1997: 162, 163). Valerie Steele is less emphatic, but acknowledges that there were avatars of the New Look in 1945 in the first collection for the Théâtre and later in 1946 Paris showings, but she regards the postwar look as 'transitional' (1997: 10). She, however, identifies sources for late-1940s fashion in the neo-Victorian fashions of the late-1930s (Steele 1991: 119). Surviving dolls indicate that aspects of the New Look were present in 1946 (as well as in the photographs of the original, lost 1945 wardrobe). Some suits and daywear – especially in the photographs of the first collection – kept the boxy, compact silhouettes of the war era and there were 'Edwardian' line dresses with slimmer skirts, flowing around the figure and featuring extremely complicated draped silhouettes, but cinched waists and bell-shaped skirts appeared throughout the collections of both 1945 and 1946, especially in eveningwear, but also in daywear.

Details too pre-empt the New Look. The romantic-styled millinery, such as wide-brimmed hats, with flowers and veiling, associated with the New Look, is clearly in place, even including some of the cowl and neckline draping details to balance the bell skirts which were a fairly standard 1950s style. The possibility that the New Look of 1947 is also a continuation of some extreme ideas of the immediate prewar years is also upheld. Balenciaga's black wool dress coat in the Théâtre, with a heavy bow detail around the hips, continues the Victorian-style flowing skirts and tight-waisted lines of his prewar 'Infanta' style dresses. This Balenciaga coat inspired a similar garment in white for doll collectors in the Gene range in the late-1990s, but the designer was uncredited. Perhaps only the heavy emphasis and weighting of the platform-styled shoes indicates a distinct difference from the look of a few years ahead. Whilst Dior's name does not actually appear in the Théâtre de la Mode, his ideas are generally ascribed to the contributions of the Lucien LeLong house for which he then worked. One of the artists involved in the backdrops, Georges Geoffroy, was Dior's colleague and was closely associated with Dior's art-based activities in the 1930s (Charles-Roux 1991b: 166).

The Théâtre has never travelled to Australia, but the same year that it was sent to America, a selection of actual garments from 1946 showings was sent out to Australia and paraded in gala events at major department stores by visiting French mannequins on tour with the clothes (Mitchell 1994a: 42–3). In a country where the local population was controlled by rationing and coupons, the collection appeared delightful and unreal. Many designers in the 1946 Australian parades such as Carven, Fath and LeLong also featured in the Théâtre de la Mode. Surviving newsreel films in the Australian National Film and Sound Archives of these parades show the same luxurious precursors of the New Look as were seen in the Théâtre de la Mode: the sweeping skirts, cinched waists and nostalgic, sumptuous vision of dress. These 1946 Australian showings, whilst obscure in an international context of the history of fashion, due to being preserved on film provide valuable cross-reference to the Théâtre de la Mode as a demonstration of the strength of French couture prior to the emergence of the New Look.

Fashion marketing did not entirely forget the Théâtre in the postwar years, although it had lapsed into obscurity by the 1980s. Alice Early provides a tantalising account – not repeated by any other writer on dolls – of another collection of doll-sized French Haute Couture of the postwar era. This collection graced what Early describes in general terms as the first international congress for man-made textile fibres in 1954 and was a retrospective of the past half century of French couture. In some cases companies provided miniatures of their most successful designs and in other cases companies worked from photographs and documentary evidence representing a particular era. 'Every fashion was represented, every occasion was provided for – garden parties, race meetings, dances, opera and theatre parties, sports wear as worn from 1900 to the present day [i.e. 1954]' (Early

1955: 166). In this case, an animated parade was provided by the puppets of the avant-garde Yves Joly puppet troupe, one of the most renowned and innovative in immediate postwar Europe. The governing impetus here was not political expedience and the shadow of war, but the intense efforts being made by the synthetic-fibre industry to obtain the cooperation of the French couture industry.

The Théâtre also inspired a smaller tribute from British designers in 1954, who dressed a doll called Virginia. She was even supplied with modern hosiery and cosmetics in doll-sized packages (Early 1955: 167). Virginia was the star of a large exhibition of dolls raising funds for the Greater London Fund for the Blind (Eaton 2001: 26), attracting widespread press attention in Britain and overseas (Anon 1954: 19). From early photographs Virginia was modelled in either ceramic or wax, as she is more delicate than the hard plastic dolls that were the staple of British postwar manufacture. In her refined features and the balletic precision and poise of her arms and hands, Virginia consciously echoed 1950s canons of fashion photography. As different images from the 1950s show her standing and seated, she resembled a doll rather than a clothes stand or a store dummy, to the degree that she is flexibly jointed.

Adult Novelties and Grotesque Dolls of the 1920s and 1930s

To track this lineage of fashion dolls during the period 1900–1950, one skirts the universal presence of dolls in adult life of the 1920s. If dolls were linked to mainstream art and design in the interwar years the links operated not so much through elegance and high style but through a range of sentiments of grotesquerie, whimsy and novelty, which had a modernist – if comical – impetus, in their movement towards simplifying and abstracting form and design; they also over-turned formal and decorous hierarchies, although they did not share modernism's sense of gravitas and mission. Dolls and doll-like figures, sometimes called 'half dolls' as they were made in porcelain or wax to the waist with lower bodies made from a variety of materials, abounded in the 1920s, as did fabric and papier mâché boudoir dolls dressed as everything from Hollywood starlets to eighteenth-century *bergères*. Dolls lounged publicly in fashionable interiors, in drawing rooms as well as bedrooms. In the shape of powder bowls, perfume flaçons and pincushions they decorated women's dressing tables. Topping crocheted milk jug covers, they were an essential and fashionable item in interwar Australia to keep the flies out of the milk and beverages at elegant garden parties and tea parties. Larger porcelain and wax dolls hid telephones under their voluminous skirts. Some had lightbulbs inserted under silk panniers and crinolines to be used as lamps. Other dolls spun around on gramophone turntables and performed innumerable weird, wonderful and novelty activities around social life in the 1920s, hitherto hardly known to either doll or human. The many functions of dolls in adult life of the 1920s are summed up by a 1923 advertisement for the Italian Lenci dolls from *Playthings*, the North American toy trade journal, located by John Noble. 'Buy a Lenci doll to place on a cassock, to lend colour to your boudoir, to decorate a corner of your limousine' (qtd Noble 1999: 18). These novelties were a vernacular expression of the vastly different outlook and experience of postwar society, and the supersession of the moods and demeanour of the Edwardian and Victorian eras. I will split hairs and suggest that these doll-like figures were not fashion dolls per se; their function was not that of being an interlocutor between dolls, high fashion and the general public, although they themselves had a popularity informed by fashion's seasonal changes.

Many of these dolls which had such a strong presence in adult life in the 1920s were related to the new artform of animation, and to popular graphics in the print media. As such, their pedigree pre-dates the First World War with Rose O'Neill's famous Kewpie dolls, modelled in bisque after her stylised humourous illustrations for several years before the war. These novelties also highlight the arrival of the cartoon series in the newspapers and various forms of dolls with exaggerated, grotesque styling in the early-twentieth century, quite alien to the French fashion dolls. They included the big-eyed 'googly' dolls, which enjoyed popularity leading up to the First World War, and the dolls based upon Wilhelm Busch's *Max and Moritz* stories; Busch was himself an *Urvater* of the cartoon. The pedigree of such novelty dolls stretches forward to the long-legged floppy clown dolls of the late-1960s, who also appeared publicly in adult-identified spaces and rooms of the home, the plethora of cheap porcelain dolls of the 1980s and onwards used as decorator pieces, available in every shopping mall, as well as groovy 1960s and 1970s novelties such as the Liddle Kiddles, Flatsy and the Blythe dolls.

Sometimes the dolls themselves were fashionable novelties. During the 1920s there were various crazes among adults for carrying and holding mascots and dolls. Amongst the dolls that had a life as fashion accessories were long-legged boudoir dolls, the felt Lenci dolls from Italy (who were seen as signs of modernism) and the similar French dolls such as those made by the Venus or Raynal companies in felt and other fabrics, as well as items such as muffs, handbags and purses with doll or teddy bear heads and faces, not all of which were intended for children's use. Dolls became popular as adult fashion accessories in 1921 (Coleman et al. 1986: 266), although even in 1919 'big, grown up girls' were 'craziest about these attractive toys' and 'all the returning officers are bearing gifts of these delectable dolls to their sweethearts, wives and mothers . . .' (*Toys and Novelties*, 1919; qtd Coleman et al. 1986: 950). 'Long limbed expensive dolls with wardrobes of fine clothes were popular in Paris' during 1927 according to the Colemans (1986: 438).

These dolls for adults were seen as descendants of wartime dolls, such as the good luck mascots worn during bombing raids and the rag dolls sold for patriotic

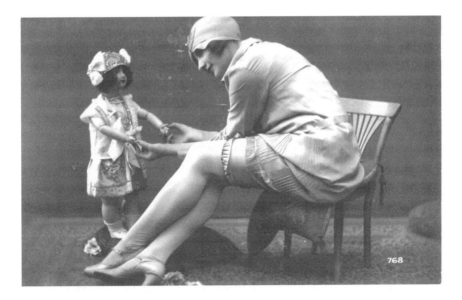

Figure 5.3 Woman with bisque doll in 1920s fashion, unidentified French postcard 1920s.

and charity fundraising (*Toys and Novelties*, 1919; qtd Coleman et al. 1986: 950). Max von Boehn saw the public carrying of dolls during the 1920s as a disturbing and vapid influence from North America. German women, by comparison, were more restrained and kept their many dolls inside the home as interior decoration features, rather than taking them outside as fashion accessories (von Boehn 1966: 218). 'Doll balls', where every guest arrived with a doll in his or her arms, were apparently the *dernier cri* in 1928 London (Coleman et al. 1986: 956). Social events throughout the 1920s frequently had a childish spin to them, such as the Baby Party where guests dressed as infants and toddlers. Such entertainments were popular throughout the decade.

Established popular fads, cartoon characters such as Bonzo the Dog, Felix the Cat and, later, Mickey Mouse reproduced in all manner of materials, joined the public presence of dolls in the 1920s as an everyday version of the infantile values that strongly informed the Dada movement's rejection of ideals of imperial citizenship and maturity, which had sent thousands to their deaths just a few years earlier. Childlike elements in 1920s fashion, such as the short skirts and the simple lines express a similarly wilful rejection of the adult. In blurring the boundaries between adulthood and the nursery, 1920s dolls again faintly reflect the conscious destabilising gestures of avant-garde art, Dada and Surrealism.

Dolls' presence in modern French life in the 1920s was reflected by their frequent inclusion in mildly erotic postcards (see Figure 5.3). Although these images are clearly produced to serve the needs of (presumed) male titillation, they

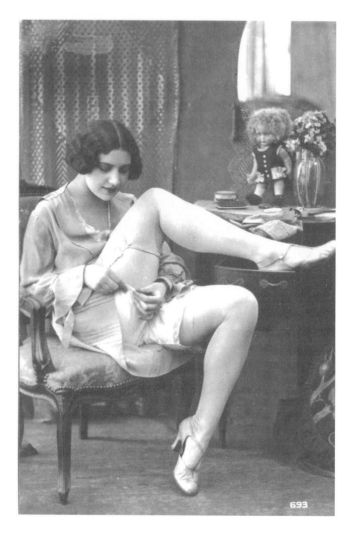

Figure 5.4 Woman with rag doll on dressing table, possibly by Venus or Raynal unidentified French postcard 1920s.

also suggest something of the intriguing power that 1920s fashion held for contemporary observers as a sign of the modern. French novelty dolls of the 1920s take their place amongst an oeuvre of better-known indicators of modernity and fashionable change in women's appearance such as short skirts, *garçonne* styling, Mary Jane shoes, cloche hats and Marcel waves. Clown and pierrot dolls are especially seen in erotic postcards, but the fancy Raynal and Venus rag dolls with wild perms and cartoon-like face painting also appear (see Figure 5.4). Raynal and Venus were both esteemed French manufacturers of modernist rag dolls in the

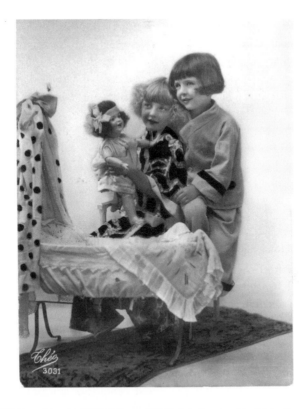

Figure 5.5 Two girls with SFBJ doll mould 236, tinted postcard by Chéo, France 1920s.

interwar era. Bisque dolls were restyled as modern women in shift dresses, despite the fact that their joints do not always accommodate the new fashions. A large bisque doll on a postcard that wears a detailed reduction of 1920s evening wear with sequinned decorations, long necklaces and a cloche hat can be ascribed with confidence to the SFBJ (see Figure 5.3). The rare surviving child dolls in such elaborate adultwear (rather than children's fashions) generally bear the trademarks of that company. A similar conflation of modernity, eroticism and dolls is seen in newsreels publicly distributed to show new underwear styles in the 1920s and 1930s, in which live models hold boudoir dolls. French postcards used as greeting cards by children and girls in France and other European countries such as Belgium and the Netherlands during the 1920s also show a similar linkage between the doll and modern fashion (see Figure 5.5).

The novelty dolls also relate to the extreme edge of the German doll reform movement. Whereas most German 'reformed' dolls were highly maternal in their intended function and spoke of citizenship and public psychological health, there was an 'expressionist', sexually explicit fantasy subgroup of non-childish dolls.

Remarkably Max von Boehn saw these sensuous dolls as belonging to the doll reform movement as much as the dolls delivering norms of appropriate psychological function into childhood (1966: 218–25). He did not censure them for their decadence or obvious modernity, marking a clear and approved incursion of the liberal and libertarian into the more expected nationalist impetus of his text. These radical dolls discussed by von Boehn include sophisticated anti-maternal dolls such as the Beardsleyesque wax dolls of Lotte Pritzel, which embody the decadence and sexual ambiguity that is popularly linked to the Weimar Republic by later twentieth-century cultural fantasies. Rainer Maria Rilke wrote an appreciation of Pritzel's dolls in 1913 (Rilke 1994: 26–39). Sadly, few of Pritzel's dolls survive outside of illustrations. They were made of fragile and vulnerable materials such as wax and silk chiffon. Idris Parry, in explaining Pritzel's work to a later audience and when annotating Rilke's appreciation, notes that the dolls' gestures, stance and style were widely imitated by dancers and stage performers during the Weimar Republic (1994: 26–7). Pritzel's epicene adult dolls do not express the sentimental prettiness that has ensured success with North American collectors during the twentieth century. '[T]hey experience no decline in their permanent sensuality . . . It is as if they yearned for a beautiful flame, to throw themselves into it like moths . . .' attested Rilke (1994: 39). Few of the creations to be seen on the pages of the current *Doll Reader* or *Contemporary Doll Collector* would express such a decadently self-destructive and extreme wish. This adult approach to dollmaking has not greatly been revived in the late-twentieth century, or at least not in the public arena of doll collectors' magazines. Pritzel, although little known to art historians, made a contribution to avant-garde art, as well as dollmaking. A friend of the Surrealist artist Hans Bellmer, she was married to the doctor treating Bellmer's wife, and provided an important influence on the artist. Together Pritzel and Bellmer pursued an interest in early dolls through visiting doll displays in German museums during the 1920s and 1930s (Taylor 2000: 71; Webb and Short 1985: 21). Pritzel's feline and exotic doll creations informed Bellmer's aesthetic and he shared his dolls as works in progress with Pritzel.

One can draw a firm line between the serious function of either the Princesses' dolls of 1938, with their portrayal of fashion as the identity and political survival of France, or the Théâtre de la Mode of 1945, with a similarly important purpose of proclaiming the survival of the French state and its most characteristic and beloved industry and the 1920s novelty dolls that have no specific function to fulfil in relation to the French fashion and textile industry. The novelty dolls do play a role in relation to the survival and trafficking of late-twentieth-century style in a more general sense. They represent the beginning of branding and character merchandising, and the 'collectable' market, of course an arena in which dolls in the late-twentieth century have featured prominently; as such the 1920s figurals, dolls and mascots are perhaps the annunciatory angels of popular culture.

In the Thrall of the Dress – Dolls, Glamour and Female Image in the 1950s

If you grew up in the 1950s you are likely to be in the thrall of the dress. We may not wear dresses any more, but we are infected by the dream dress and it erupts in the art that we make. Perhaps because we grew up with mothers who wore proper dresses with form fitting bodices, scooped necks and capped sleeves and below the fullest of full skirts, a gathering, that swirled and twirled, whizzy skirts that performed a dance of their own. We hid behind these voluminous skirts when strangers came to the door, sheltered by the New Look.

Suzanne Spunner 'The Thrall of the Dress' (1999: 14)

If you grew up female in the 1950s and 1960s, you grew up with the notion that your adult life would be glamorous, exciting and full of handsome, rich men. All vying for a chance to sweep you off your feet and marry you, so that you could live happily ever after. That was the idea presented to us in a genre of movies that we watched over and over again. Stars like Audrey Hepburn, Marilyn Monroe, Lauren Bacall, Betty Grable, Lana Turner, in movies like *Roman Holiday*, *Sabrina*, *How to Marry a Millionaire* gave us a taste of what beauty, high fashion and the right man could do for us. And what more could we want out of life?

Karen Caviale 'Playing Dress-Up With Barbie' (1997: 37)

In the wake of the dramatic launch of Dior's New Look in 1947 widespread popular curiosity in the English-speaking world about Parisian couture flourished in the late-1940s and 1950s. Despite early resistance, such as the Little Below the Knee club in the United States, a popular conception developed, from that first iconic moment, which defined French high fashion as an ideal to which all women aspired. French fashion was regarded as beautiful, quintessentially desirable and worthy of emulation, even by women who could never afford to purchase original garments. Parisian high fashion appeared at all levels of North American culture: television with *I Love Lucy*, film with *Funny Face*, 1958, and high literature with Paul Gallico's *Mrs Harris Goes to Paris*, the story of the creation and ultimate immolation of a Dior evening dress. Valerie Steele records that even children's books such as *Eloise Goes to Paris* presented Paris as the city of style (Levinthal 1998: 7). 'The late-1940s and 1950s was a time of intense interest in Paris Fashion and it was a period when the moderately priced market was flooded with fashion derivative of Paris' (Mitchell 1994b: 10). The prestige attached to fashionable imagery inspired by and sourced from French designers had a strong follow-on effect in the doll industry. The mystique of high fashionable style in the 1950s encouraged the development of the so-called 'teenage dolls' in the USA including Madame Alexander's Cissy, Aranbee's Coty Girl and Vogue Doll Company's Jill. Other names for these dolls are 'glamour dolls', 'fashionable ladies' or 'fashion dolls'. The genre is generally accepted as having been launched in 1955 by Madame Alexander's Cissy. These dolls were different to the juvenile norm accepted by the toy trade. They had moulded breasts, feet shaped to wear high-heeled shoes and large ready-made wardrobes for purchase by the doll owner. These wardrobes stressed an up-to-date, desirable fashion image and highlighted glamorous and formal clothes and accessories above the everyday. Garments made for these dolls included formal taffeta and silk dresses, handbags, real furs, appropriate jewellery and detailed hats, blocked and moulded with the same techniques and handwork as adult millinery, trimmed with veilings, flowers and feathers.

The return of the celebration of high fashion in a doll-sized format only serves to indicate the relative disappearance of the high fashion doll as a commercial product in the previous half century. The location of this revival is unexpected. The reappearance of the fashion doll as a commercial product is not amongst the original creators of Haute Couture, the French, but amongst its most enthusiastic customers, the Americans. The adult and teenage fashion dolls of the 1950s – the so-called glamorous or fashionable ladies –could be best understood as a popular reaction to the emergence of the New Look in 1947 and Dior's iconic innovations in high fashion. As such they deserve attention from fashion historians.

These adult dolls celebrate the essential characteristics of high Parisian fashion in the late-1940s and 1950s, as broadly understood by an international audience in the wake of Dior: the romantic approach to fashion design, the focus upon the evening gown with its nostalgic shape and textures, the fascination with romantic and detailed fabrics such as brocades and lace net. The dresses of the best 1950s lady dolls fully grasp the essentials of contemporary Haute Couture because not only do they obviously look backwards but they also engage with present and future technologies. They dramatically rework Victorian canons with striking contrasts of textures and scale and employ new materials, especially nylon net, to create the crinoline effects. The light shoes so popular in the era, with their arching soles and stiletto heels, proclaim the simultaneous modernity of elements of the 1950s fashion, through their employment of new technologies and materials. Nothing that a historically alert eye may expect from the look of the late-1940s and 1950s seems to be missing in the dressing and presentation of these dolls. The overall effect is enhanced by careful attention to coordination of accessories, elaborate fake flowers on corsages and hats, the careful placement of jewellery – mostly in faux pearls and diamanté. When in pristine condition, the dolls also effectively present the ideals of female grooming and cosmetics favoured during the period. A doll's 'perm' or her French roll, if not wrecked by the hands of children past, remains crisp and orderly. Paintwork replicates the formalised make-up, clearly artificial in its visibility (again a point of difference from the Victorian ideals that informed 1950s fashion design) and controlled in its flawlessness with the plucked and defined eyebrows and deep red lipstick. The plastic dolls' loyalty to the New Look silhouette creates a touching aura around these miniature, unauth-orised tributes. One only need see Sweet Sue Sophisticate in her sweeping fuchsia tulle evening dress with dramatic black velvet bow details, originally sold as the *American Beauty* dress, to recall the presence of the quintessential Dior evening dress.

These new fashion dolls were sometimes associated with the grooming that was seen as essential to the formalised female personal stylising and self-performance of the 1950s. Two of the most famous lady dolls of the 1950s, Miss Revlon and the Coty Girl, both advertised major cosmetic firms. This cross marketing of beauty aids gave a commercial impetus to overriding the advocates of the reformed, psychologically 'correct' dolls that had developed in the interwar period. Even certain domestic little girl and child dolls of the postwar period were intended to bring to mind beauty regimes and the necessity – both consumerist and social – of maintaining such regimes. Manufacturers of generic little girl dolls of medium quality often packaged their dolls with actual bottles of various beauty lotions. Most famous of all these cosmetic tie-in dolls were the Toni dolls associated with the widely advertised 'home perm'. The dolls were intended to provide girls with practice in styling hair. Likewise American cosmetics firm Harriet Hubbard Ayer was promoted through an Ideal doll in 1953. Like the Toni doll she was intended to be for 'hair play' and represented a little girl, not the adult females who would actually be buying and using cosmetics and setting lotions at home. Ironically many Toni dolls and other dolls who were marketed to be home permed and otherwise experimented on by their owners are now too damaged for collectors who seek a pristine example. Such dolls who advertised beauty products did not induct young girls into maternalism as much as provide a grass roots understanding of the obligations of high fashion, and an apprenticeship to its rituals. Later the manufacture of the Toni doll would change from Ideal to American Character Doll Corporation. This reassignment of the licence brought a new identity and persona. With the glamorous Sweet Sue Sophisticate as prototype, the Toni doll grew to resemble the product's adult consumers.

The link between dolls and the marketing of cosmetics references those texts by Baudelaire and Beerbohm which praised woman insofar as she is rendered artifi-cial by fashion and cosmetics. If Baudelaire likens woman to a strange pagan idol

(Steele 1999: 87), one can even find a doll analogy in the North American children's classic of the 1930s, *Hitty* by Rachel Field, in which a doll reflecting white ideals of beauty finds herself being used somewhere during the mid-nineteenth century as a pagan idol by a tribe of 'South Seas Islanders' (Field 1947: 69–72). This image of Pacific Otherness and its appearance in a children's book is a curious by-product of the writings of Margaret Mead, and others, in which island life promises a guilt-free sexuality and condones the permissiveness of the 1920s. Hitty assures her readers that she does not lose her chemise, even as she is set upon the temple altar and worshipped. Yet her adventure is ratified by the writings of Baudelaire. Woman, he proclaimed, 'is a kind of idol stupid perhaps but dazzling' (qtd Steele 1999: 87). All women could therefore be dolls. Cosmetics indicated her confected, artificial nature.

If one could trace an ambiguity in using play dolls styled as little girls to encourage the purchase and usage of chemical products substantially intended for adult consumption, then cosmetic manufacturers themselves seemed to be unsure of quite where these advertising dolls should be placed and whom they addressed. One account suggests that Charles Revson, president of Revlon cosmetics, did not quite see how the Miss Revlon doll fitted his company's profile, but found the royalties generated by the use of the brandname 'Revlon' for a best-selling doll most acceptable (Izen 2001: 103–4). The Ideal Doll company drove the Miss Revlon concept and she was originally intended to be part of a larger series of advertising tie-ins with various branches of the beauty and fashion industries. For example Ideal planned for doll-sized foundation garments for Miss Revlon, bearing popular brandnames of adult underwear such as Formfit (Izen 2001: 103–4). These garments were not actually put into production but again this cross-marketing indicates the role played by the glamorous adult doll as training for the maintenance of a feminine and fashionable self. The advertising for the doll proclaims:

> Your Revlon doll is different – different in many ways to any other doll in the world. She looks like the beautiful girl in the famous Revlon cosmetics – with her peaches and cream expression and the prettiest shades of lips and nails. So beautiful because she has learned the real Revlon beauty secrets. That's why we call her the Revlon doll – because Revlon means beauty. (Anon c.late-1950s)

Barbie's titanic level of fame, the cultural legends that have gathered around her and the long bibliography of analytical studies and fanzines have erased the complex cultural histories of the lady dolls of the 1950s, the glamorous lady dolls who were her obvious precursors. She should rightfully be classed as a related phenomenon to these glamour dolls, and they should be the subject of the same type of cultural analysis that has been so fruitfully directed to Barbie. The glamour dolls proved that high fashion as ubiquitous sign of the feminine could be translated into a doll size, and Barbie arrived at the end of half a decade of exploration of a high fashion image as presented in doll form in North America during the mid-to late-1950s.

However, Barbie also drew upon the simultaneous appearance in 1955 of another modern adult-personaed doll: the West German Bild Lilli doll, who was based upon a popular cartoon character in the *Bild* newspaper. Thus there are two converging genealogies for Barbie in the 1950s, an American and a German: two dolls, Bild Lilli and Madame Alexander's Cissy. The American side of this dual history witnessed the return of the adult fashion doll as staple product in the 1950s, thus providing a market niche for Barbie. Her physical format and appearance have a close connection with the German Lilli. Behind both streams of Barbie's history stands the French fashion doll of the nineteenth century. Both Cissy and Bild Lilli referenced the Parisienne as adult female reduced to a small-scale commodity. These two cultural phenomena – Barbie's twin pedigrees – commenced around the same time, but ran in separate directions until they were united with the production of the Barbie doll. The American lineage of Barbie is most obviously linked to fashion's history and rituals, but the German side of the Barbie story references the general culture of the female image of the 1950s. In turn high fashion is itself such a celebrated and central exemplar of the construction of femininity during the 1950s that both sides of Barbie's genealogy respond to the centrality of fashion in the female experience of the 1950s.

Barbie's Predecessors: the European Story

The German ancestress of the Barbie doll, Bild Lilli, usually known simply as Lilli, highlights the complex positioning of the feminine in the 1950s. She is a point at which doll history intersects with wider cultural and political experience. Lilli positions Barbie and dolls generally in the heartlands of late-twentieth-century popular historical obsessions. Frequently the Bild Lilli doll is reduced to meaning nothing but sex and cheap provocation. Laura Meissner, writing in the North American doll collectors' magazine *Millers Magazine*, emphasised the risqué elements of Lilli as sophisticated and positive values, celebrating her as the 'femme fatale' of the dollworld. For Meissner Lilli changed the world of the fashion doll forever from 'demure to femme fatale' (1997: 64). This image of Lilli has captured attention and was inspired by M.G. Lord's *Forever Barbie*. Both popular history (Miller 1998: 68–9) and academic literature (Dubin 1999: 20; Ockman 1999: 78; Rand 1995: 32–7) claim that Barbie 'cleaned up' a men's sex novelty. Perhaps such representations of the transition from Lilli to Barbie affirm the curative aspects of North American civilisation over an older but more sordid 'Europe', but Lilli speaks of far broader issues. Lord does not see the process in these racist and reductive terms, but other writers use Lilli to seek to emphasise the strangeness of 'Germany' or even 'Europe' – that is friend and foe alike – against North America as norm.

G.Wayne Miller in *Toy Wars*, sees Lilli guilelessly and crudely as a direct symbol of the Otherness of culture and behaviour of the 'Germans'.

> Her appeal to German-speaking men, who kept her in their cars or used her as a sexual come-on to randy girl friends, was her tight sweaters and short skirts, which could be removed. (Miller 1998: 68)

Curiously here the clothes that indicate foolishness or excess in the hands of women and fashion as a sign of women's unsuitability for public life now, when placed in the hands of men, represent sexual availability. However, specifically 'German-speaking men' are indicated, for what would 'normal' men be doing with a doll? Likewise equally grotesque and un-American are their 'randy' girlfriends. The doll Lilli clearly indicates why the Germans are 'not us'. Lilli/Barbie is possibly another expression of why the reiteration of the German double defeat of 1918 and 1945 eternally fascinates popular culture. Beyond human rights issues, these two defeats were a punitive retaliation for the Germans' misfortune not to be born as one of 'us' and also for their a priori strangeness.

The very title of Miller's book, *Toy Wars The Epic Struggle Between G.I. Joe, Barbie and the Companies who Made Them*, indicates military conflict between the home-grown and admirable 'GI Joe' and the alien Other – Barbie being short, as Lord reminds us, for 'Barbarian' (1994: 43). Even academics use Lilli to indicate the strange behaviours of 'Germans'. 'Unlike Barbie, Lilli was not made for children but for men who displayed her on the dashboard of their cars and, more bizarre still, gave her to their girlfriends instead of flowers or chocolates' (Ockman 1999: 78).[1] If Barbie's source in Lilli is not used to define her as a symbol of the 'German', with the memory of La Barbarina, Barbara Campanini, a ballet dancer and one of the very few women in whom Frederick the Great seemed to show any emotional interest, Barbie's own name still has clear links to German military tradition. Barbie is an extremely troubling symbol of the German who so far stands undefeated, and therefore stands against the general popular cultural meaning of the 'German'.

M.G. Lord, in particular, fleshes out this popular cultural tradition in which Lilli/Barbie stands as a symbol of German history. She likens Lilli to Fassbinder's Maria Braun, as a Germania in disguise who suffers/survives her nation's humiliation and eventual economic rebirth (1994: 28–9). Lilli is 'the vanquished Aryan gold digging her way back to posterity' (1994: 29). Lord casts Lilli further into modern German history, pondering whether Barbie may have had a previous life during the Second World War when, dressed in a glittering black evening dress, she sang in 'some smoky Berlin Cabaret . . . the depths of an Axis-power cocktail lounge'. The evening dress was described as 'very Dietrich, evocative of the chanteuse she portrayed in Billy Wilder's *Foreign Affair*'. 'One could imagine the Lilli doll . . . rasping out *Falling in Love Again*' (1994: 48). The dark glamour of a smoke-filled lounge peopled by Axis officers is a confected image of a German past based upon popular images drawn from filmic interpretations of the Weimar Republic and the Second World War, which frequently conflate the visual imagery of the two eras. Considering the misogyny of the Nazi era, it is ironic that Lilli/ Barbie is so frequently read as a sign of the Third Reich in popular culture. Despite her public record of visibly performed anti-Nazism, Marlene Dietrich's Lola Lola persona, her dressing and stage mannerisms have been recast as a sign of the nascent Third Reich in films such as *Cabaret*, 1972, and *The Damned*, 1969, and this symbolism has passed into popular currency.

Lilli/Barbie's symbolic performance is not without precedent. The permutations of the Isherwood/Weimar Republic 'Cabaret' theme from short story to stage to film to stage to film as musical and back again to the stage demonstrate how German culture and political life are persistently characterised by the centre and the left in English-speaking countries as queer and feminine/feminised (Mizejewski 1992; Peers 2001: 45–6). The pattern can be taken back even further to the turn of the century with the figure of Kaiser Wilhelm II, who was imaged as being about performance, spectatorship, the modern media and a sexuality that was different/ indefinable/ambiguous (Peers 2001: 43–56). If, as Linda Mizejewski and others suggest, the metaphorical image of war between Germany and America was a conflict between essentialism/purity and surface appearance/performance, then Barbie brings fashion into this key postmodernist equation. Barbie, women and Germany all represent strangeness, the *unheimlich* and artificial. What seem to be random or wilful links in lurid popular imaginations have a far wider resonance and cogency. There is also a practical source for these legends and fantasies. Rare surviving intact examples indicate that Bild Lilli was actually packaged and distributed in North America during the mid-1950s – prior to Barbie's launch – as Lilli Marleen, which placed her immediately within the popular culture of the Second World War.[2]

Who is Barbie, then, when Lord emphasises her transvestite body with 'broad shoulders, narrow hips and huge breasts' (1994: 14, 213–14) as well as her German origins?[3] And how did she get to America? One popular myth reported in the late-1990s on an internet site suggests that Barbie was redeemed and brought to the United States by her 'Jewish Mother', Ruth Handler. 'That the "most potent icon of American popular culture in the late twentieth century" emerged from the post-Reich demi-monde would seem ironic enough. However the little plastic Aryan tart was rescued from her Teutonic ignominy by a Jewish saviour' (Jacobson 1995).[4] Here Barbie's gender is not stated, although as a 'tart' who bonds with her mother, she would appear to be feminine. In a successful off-Broadway musical of the 1990s and later a film of cult reputation and status, *Hedwig and the Angry Inch*, 2001 (directed and written by John Cameron Mitchell with music by Stephen Trask), the transcendent blonde of Teutonic origins is neither man nor woman, but an East German soldier brought to America by a GI. This East German had suffered a botched sex-change operation which left him/her with 'the angry inch' of flesh, after which s/he named her rock band, the Angry Inch. Again we have the image of Germany as strange and queer, yet simultaneously militaristic and authoritarian, both masculine and feminine. In the lyrics Hedwig describes herself as strong and implacable like the Berlin wall: 'Don't you know me, Kansas City? I'm the new Berlin Wall. Try and tear ME down!' In the original productions Hedwig wears a cape painted to look like graffiti on the Wall. 'Yankee go home' reads one side '. . . with me' reads the other, thus subversively introducing a homosexual subtext into the morally pure narratives of the Second World War and the cold war. One notes again the trope of linking the performative/cabaret with 'German History'. Barbie seems to have been present in the London stage production of September to November 2000, which closed early after generally critical reviews,[5] if descriptions of Hedwig on stage are accurate. 'Kitted out in pink-fringed cowboy boots, stone-wash denim frock and Farrah Fawcett wig, she looks like a hybrid of Dolly Parton and Courtney Love' wrote *The Independent*, and *The Times* likewise recognised a similar style: 'The strapping Michael Cerveris certainly delivers, appearing like a cross between Dolly Parton and Courtney Love' (qtd Albemarle 2000).

A haunting poem by Denise Duhamel *Holocaust Barbie* is drawn from these popular myths linking Barbie to modern German history.

> . . . Her Aryan air, the ease in
> which her arm, unable to bend at the elbow,
> would salute. The terror when she saw a pile
> of dolls like herself, naked and dirty, in the mass grave of a toy chest.
> Barbie sought hypnotists and healers,
> who all saw the connection, though none could be sure
> whether in her past Barbie was the Nazi or the Jew.
>
> (Duhamel 1999: 163)

West German history lends an extraordinary sense of change and moment to the meaning of Lilli and therefore Barbie. Consumerism in West Germany in particular marked a physical calibration of the climb out of postwar occupation and the humiliation of defeat; the latter being a burden borne most directly by women in the most obvious of personal experience from Allied bombing of civilian towns to rape by the Red Army. Yet the specific direction of hostilities towards female bodies as much as male also indicated how women as much as men could become a de facto symbol of the state or nation in growing prosperity as well as defeat.

> Lilli's story is the story of the Fifties everywhere but particularly the Fifties in Germany. In West Germany to be precise, because Lilli was born just as the western section of a divided Germany was starting to take off economically after the devastation of World War II . . .
>
> Women's role changed dramatically in the years up to Lilli's creation. In the ten years after 1945, West German women moved from 'rubble women' clinging to survival in bombed out cities to a much more secure economic and social position. They could start to enjoy life again. Thanks to the new appliances, they had more free time. And besides their greater economic freedom, they could be more independent thanks to a 1957 law implementing the postwar constitution's promise of equal rights for women and men. (Astor-Kaiser 1999: 62)

M.G. Lord also links Lilli/Barbie to the *Wirtschaftswunder*, the rapid growth of the West German economy after the war. Lilli/Barbie was a woman who has seen 'the smouldering ruins of postwar Germany and knew the horrors that had preceded them' (1994: 35). She was certainly 'determined not to suffer again as long as there were men with cheque books' (1994: 8, 35).

Lilli/Barbie also resonates with another updated Germania as demonstrated by the German film *The Girl Rosemarie*, 1958 (directed by Rolf Thiele 1958). *Rosemarie* was a scathing political critique of postwar West German society. To indict the ethos of Adenauer's Germany through the image of a venal prostitute, Rosemarie Nitribitt, has both right-wing and left-wing resonances. As symbol Nitribitt could indicate the humiliation of defeat and 'selling out' to the money-driven United States, in addition to the left-wing critique of the power of capitalism foregrounded by director Thiele. The prostitute was identified not only as the quintessential West German, but the quintessential woman (for are not women always on their knees before the coloniser and victor?), as she desired, and gained, televisions, tape recorders, white goods and cars, materialist pleasures of good clothes and homewares. Moreover Rosemarie/Everywoman was decked out from head to toe in Haute Couture fashions. Her Mephistophelean pimp was a Frenchman. Thus he could easily tempt Rosemarie to work against her own nation and its conservative aristocratic elites, with the suave credibility lent by his Parisian sense of style and his promise to facilitate Rosemarie's remake as an exemplar of the New Look, a figure from *Vogue* or *L'Officiel*. Her French tempter was, in effect, Haute Couture and he recruited Rosemarie to fight in the war that had been going on since 1870 between France and Germany; a war that Emile-Louis Jumeau recognised as early as the 1870s could be fought with style and styling as well as bullets.

Barbie's plethora of consumer goods and her luxury open tourers are close to those amassed by Rosemarie in the film. Perhaps we may even excuse Barbie's relentless pursuit of material goods if we understand that one of her possible motivations is to obliterate a miserable past. Certainly the universal consumerism in Western countries after the war reflected the celebration of the end of wartime impositions of shortages, 'make do and mend' or ersatz. The modernist critique of bourgeois morality in the 1958 *Rosemarie* film gratifies some audiences and the film was remade in 1996 as a portentous colour version, directed by Bernd Eichinger. This remake is feminist, insofar as it portrays Rosemarie as a victim of repression and social double standards, and modernist, insofar as it unselfconsciously believes in its own Darwinist mission of cultural advancement and targets the 'bourgeois' with a retardataire fervour and virtually Stalinist two dimensionality. Both films of the Rosemarie story are marked by their inability to distance themselves from the misogynist and prejudiced values of their modernist underpinnings; this is especially striking in the case of the later remake. However, a felicitous intertextual serendipity in the later film was a reference to the Lilli doll. When the rebellious Rosemarie leaves the confines of her bourgeois home early in the remake to hitch a lift out of town and away from her narrow, repressive family,[6] her hair is dressed in the blonde ponytail associated with Lilli. Rosemarie even wears the white blouse and dark skirt of the so-called (in English) 'Hitchin' Lilli': a small plastic figurine representing Lilli hitch-hiking, which was made in West Germany as a popular dashboard ornament.

Yet Lilli's relationship to 'the war' is not only a specifically German story, nor should it be read as one of the myriad signs of German strangeness in popular cultural interpretations of 'the war' or both World Wars. The cultural myths that have sprung up around Lilli relate to a more widespread, diffused anxiety about the feminine during the mid-twentieth century. Women were seen to co-exist uncomfortably with collective wartime good in many countries. The Australian filmmaker Damien Parer explicitly preceded his Oscar-winning documentary about soldiers at war, *Kokoda Frontline*, 1942, with a homily in which he spoke directly at his female homefront audience, accusing them of being frivolous and self-centred in comparison with the honourable sacrifice being made by saintly males under fire – surely an Australian reworking of the old *Dolsch im Rück* legend of the good frontline warrior betrayed by homefront laziness and treachery. Whereas in Germany it was a left/right conflict, in Australia it was a male/female conflict, with woman betraying the soldier. Throughout the film the commentary from time to time turns away from describing the military action on screen to address an imaginary audience of women and accuse them of shrilly complaining of discomforts and hassles which were minor in comparison with those that frontline soldiers faced daily with stoicism. *Kokoda Frontline* received the first Academy Award for any Australian production, thus suggesting that the appeal of this self-righteous piece of misogyny was more than parochial.

The British response to the New Look placed female desire in express conflict with collectivising and the post war national good. Sir Stafford Cripps, British Chancellor of the Exchequer, tried to persuade the British fashion industry that it would help the economy to keep the short skirt (Gardiner 1999: 41). Colin McDowell suggests that the New Look was read as an affront to the 'egalitarianism' of the Attlee Government (1997: 171) and cites 1940s voices as diverse as 'Mabel Ridleigh, MP for North Illford, Essex', and journalist Marjorie Post raised against the lavish styling and cut (1997: 172–8). Women were seen as the more likely traitors to the collective war effort of the community. When British commentators of the 1940s believed that self-indulgent followers of fashion 'show[ed] no conscience' (qtd. 1997: 178) they placed fashionable women in explicit opposition to the suffering postwar humanity. Designers were described as 'fashion dictators' who 'curtail[ed]' the 'freedom' (qtd. 1997: 178) of their public. These were emotionally loaded words in the context of recent world events. The strange conflation of stereotypes of German/Nazi values and the beautiful woman again can be tracked through this extreme vocabulary. It was claimed in mid-1947, and therefore following the launch of the New Look, that the Salvation Army in the United States denounced current fashion as insulting Christian notions of charity (Anon 1947: 3), yet again suggesting that fashion and conforming to fashionable style was placed outside conventional notions of humanity. There is a deeper and more complex history to the hostility shown towards Barbie, other than opposition to her supposedly frivolous, specious female persona and her gluttonous capitalist consumption of clothes and consumer goods including cars and real estate. Perhaps contempt is directed at Barbie because that body clad in pink lycra could never selflessly serve the state by either providing new soldiers or submitting to potential frontline sacrifice. Even more seriously, when that body once did put itself at its nation's disposal – in a former life before the 'operation' – it wore *feldgrau* rather than khaki.

If the Second World War by changing the basic nature of conflict from a bipolar push-pull of masculine nation-state against masculine nation-state to a triangulated conflict where the aim of (rightfully) combating the Nazi regime was frequently and conveniently pursued through targeting its politically relatively disempowered female citizens, this morally ambiguous stratagem also changed women's relationship to national mythologies and the public space. The identication of civilian women as political enemies and de facto frontline soldiers, seen as early as the Spanish Civil War with such fascist actions as the bombing of Guernica,[7] having been legitimised by practice, not only exposed women to danger during the conflict but left them to carry the burdens of the state in defeat. Could women no longer be dismissed as irrelevant to the symbolic validation of the state, relegated to the background, erased from the agora or returned to a position of impotence in the symbolic hierarchy? They became central performers in the changes in public culture and experience in the postwar era. Part of the inescapable fascination of the

Barbie doll in the last four decades derives from her descent from Bild Lilli who expresses this fundamental reconstruction not only of 'Germany', but of public myth in Anglo-European culture. The visceral depth of response to the New Look and the completeness of its possession of the postwar imagination as symbol of renewal and remaking was not only due to the power of Marc Boussac's publicity machine, or even because it represented a return to plenitude after wartime privation, but because it resonated with these deep and unspoken cultural changes, and made them visible in a peerlessly stylish manner. In the Théâtre de la Mode, Jean Cocteau's tableau superimposed beautiful evening gowns over shattered timber and masonry; it made a series of contrasts (war and peace, male and female, glamour and ruins) but the juxtaposition reads as if the glorious creatures with nipped in waists and spreading skirts were femme fatales, the catalysts and queens of that physical destruction of male infrastructure.

Lilli gave solid form to postwar experience, and was an eloquent symbol of the new Germany hanging from the rear-view mirrors of trucks and flashy cars. Rather than use her tradename, older Germans still remember Lilli as the doll who hung below rear-view mirrors (Gerling 1999: 58). 'In the '50s in Germany, car mascots were very popular and were thought to bring luck in avoiding accidents' (1999: 58). Lilli's first appearance in the newspaper *Bild* indicates the new and popularist medium of tabloid newspapers that marked a different – cleansed, transformed – public spirit in West Germany and defined the capitalist character of the new society. Lilli's origins again place her as a performer of postwar change and modernity. The Lilli hitchhiking figurine, made concurrently to the dolls, was of course another sign of modern life and habits in postwar West Germany that was associated with this popular female persona.

Whilst Lilli has specific German meanings, the sense of emergence into a vastly expanded world of consumerism, leisure, household appliances and aesthetically charged clothing modes is the story of both 'women' and 'Europe' in the postwar era. A 1999 exhibition in a major German public museum, the Nürnberg Toy Museum explicitly linked Lilli not with the expected signifiers that shadow her in English language discourses even at a professional level, such as the Third Reich and sexual licence, but with a sense of expanding possibilities for women (Astor-Kaiser 1999: 60–65). Lilli evoked such postwar phenomena as the availability of new household labour-saving devices and the fascination with towering female icons across popular culture in Europe.

As Astor-Kaiser indicates (1999: 60), Lilli could join the new European cinema stars as a symbol of the expanding female experience of consumption in Europe. Such changing female paradigms also chart the emergence of a European response to American culture and the development of a European confidence in following new cultural patterns. Symbols such as Lilli and these new European stars as home-grown divas express the complex balance of cultural power between a devastated

Europe, poor in material goods and infrastructure, and the pervasive cultural influence of the United States. Yet during the 1950s there was also a counter-traffic in popular culture from Europe towards North America. High fashion, low fashion, 'Capri' pants, matador pants, espadrilles, foreign language cinema, European film stars and songs like *Volare, Amore, Arriverderci Roma*, the *Happy Wanderer* (an unexpected international hit record) and, of course, even the Lilli doll, both as herself and as Barbie, travelled from Europe to acquire iconic status in North America.

Amongst the figures who expanded postwar experiences of the feminine Astor-Kaiser specifically names Brigitte Bardot and Sophia Loren as symbols of the new European woman of the 1950s. One could also add Simone Signoret, Anna Magnani, Alida Valli and Gina Lollobrigida as other European film actresses beloved by international audiences. Lilli was understood by her original audience in such terms. An early German advertisement quoted by Peggie Gerling asked rhetorically whether Lilli was 'created after – Monroe, Lollo or Sophia' (1999: 59). These screen sirens could be identified as feminist figures of possibility rather than exploited figures only providing voyeuristic fulfilment to men. Through the cinema such European stars not only spread an image of sexual allure, but of style and glamour. They instructed women by articulating a new sense of public confidence and forthrightness. While undoubtedly sexual/sexualised by the distinctly (and still undeconstructed) male patterns of auteurship in much postwar European cinema, these women were also larger than life and resourceful in the face of ubiquitous male power. These towering female personae culminated in the poster goddess in evening dress played by Anita Eckberg, who came to life to haunt a mean-spirited Italian bureaucrat in Fellini's *Temptation of Dr Antonio*, one of the short films of the Italian filmed anthology *Boccaccio '70* (1962). The *Temptation* clearly linked sheer transcendent female beauty with the newness of modern life, customs and advertising. Whereas frequently advertising and consumerism are read by commentators as rendering women powerless, through employing demeaning stereotypes and duping its targeted audience by overcoming their prudence, the *Temptation* indicated that modern images of women in advertising had a deeper, timeless resonance with classical archetypes. The mystic power of Fellini's billboard goddess resonates with M.G. Lord's identification of Barbie as a modern incarnation of an ancient fertility goddess (1994: 74–9) and shares Barbie's sense of high fashionable style. Do those who decry Barbie's supposedly tawdry sexuality in fact deeply fear the imperium of her irresistible sexual allure, or fear the image of woman unfettered and transcendent? These European stars were living demonstrations on the screen in small towns and villages across many nations that women could demand pleasure, clothes, appearance, sexual fulfilment. Hitherto proper family life, not only in Nazi Germany, had expected women to deny personal desires and ambitions in their role as moral guide and spiritual power within the family, whilst public culture validated male experience.

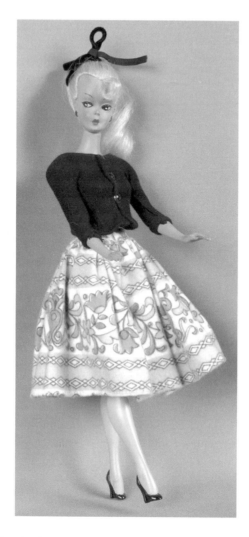

Figure 6.1 Bild Lilli, sculpted by Reinhard Beuthien and Max Weissbrodt in original skirt and jumper by Martha Maar c.1955, image by courtesy of McMasters Harris Auctions, USA.

Despite G.Wayne Miller highlighting the strangeness and inferred perversion of the German men who bought Lilli (1998: 68), Peggie Gerling suggests that girls and women raised Lilli into a cult object. Teenagers and children began buying her in large quantities as a toy, whereas men used her to hang inside the windscreens of cars and trucks or attach her to their dashboards. Young West German girls' colonisation of this adult mascot made the production of innumerable fashionable dresses for Lilli economically viable (Gerling 1999: 58–9). This new opportunity to buy a collection of dresses for Lilli had many cultural meanings. The option of being able to buy a range of ready-made clothing presented the real possibility of shopping till one dropped, unencumbered by rationing. Shopping until one dropped overwrote dropping dead due to wartime conflict. Lilli's wardrobe is, like that of her American contemporary Miss Revlon, an index of middle-class dressing. Lilli went in two slightly different directions to her glamorous American doll peers. Her clothes were mostly designed by Martha Maar (Gerling 1999: 58), a veteran of the prewar doll trade for many decades, director of the 3M doll company. Maar provided Lilli with a number of pretty frilly dresses in prints, including 1950s interpretations of *tracht* and *dirndls*, Southern German and Tyrolean peasant dress – a look that found many adherents among women and teenage girls outside Germany as well as within, in dresses with faux bodices or corselets over frilly white underblouses. Additionally, more than other fashionable dolls of the 1950s, Lilli favoured various informal fashions in women's pants, Capris and exaggeratedly tiny shorts; the shorts inspired one of Barbie's early fashions *Vacation Time*, 1965. Lilli's dresses were often a little shorter than the fashionable length of the 1950s to expose her beautifully sculpted legs. These legs in turn were the exact model for the early Barbie.

Lilli's middle-class clothing found favour not only in Germany but also elsewhere in Europe, including Italy and Scandinavia, where she was distributed and sold as a child's toy. She was not only a toy doll or a sex novelty, but her fashions were enjoyed for their own sake. A German fashion doll may seem to be the toyworld's ultimate oxymoron, but in the *Wirtschaftswunder* years of the 1950s German fashion apparently attracted more serious international attention beyond the domestic market than it had in living memory. Such was the claim of an Australian journal article, which made an interesting distinction: Paris might set the ideal, but West German fashion more accurately anticipated how women actually wore the styles as the season developed (Anon 1952b: 52).

Bild Lilli's ready-made trousseau re-established the idea that one could buy dresses and accessories from Jenny Béreux's long-forgotten boutique for dolls in Paris. Throughout the late-twentieth century this idea of the doll's ever-expanding trousseau, changing and reflecting each new seasonal development, has often been assumed to be characteristic of Barbie alone. The economic demands of this growing trousseau and the supposedly 'bad' lessons that it teaches about consumerism are frequently ascribed to Barbie's malign influence. In fact the widespread designing and supply of ready-made clothes was well established by the end of the 1950s simultaneously by the German Lilli and the American fashion dolls. These 1950s doll fashions revived the idea of the French ateliers supplying trousseaus for dolls, but followed the updated format of ready-made massmarket clothing. Ready-made clothes also removed doll dressing from lessons in domestic economy: no longer did diligent Suzettes make clothes for their Bleuettes, but they bought them ready-made for Lilli. If there were voices, especially radical voices, who decried the materialistic optimism of the 1950s, then woman, as the customer explicitly addressed in the 1950s discourses of marketing and product development, was also castigated.

That Lilli can be read simultaneously as a trollop and as a figure of self-realisation is part of a wider pattern of deep fissures in the contradictory meanings ascribed to the feminine in the 1950s. This complex mix of limitation and liberation, of maternity and allure, of pleasure versus duty, of self-surveillance and maintenance, of the simultaneous circulation of belittling, reductive images of women and monumental fixations on certain deified female personae, from Queen Elizabeth II to Marilyn Monroe, predisposes fashion to be a particularly apt and memorable symbol of the 1950s. Not only has the superb, dramatic presence of the best 1950s Haute Couture singled out fashion as perhaps one of the most clear and obvious signs of the 1950s, but the multilayered and flexible nature of fashion amongst the arts recommended it to later generations as the quintessential symbol of this complex decade. Dior's New Look, though certainly romantic and nostalgic in its vocabulary, could be read concurrently as a potent symbol of revolution, but the impetus of the greatest change was not carried by the expected revolutionary hero – the man – but by women. The famous image of Parisian working-class housewives tearing New Look dresses off young women not only indicated the misogyny that is, for some, inherent in Dior's stylised imagery of the feminine and closely recalled the recent, similar visible ritual of the public humiliation of the *collaborateuses*, but also capitalised on a realisation that certain (privileged) women were refusing the narrow and servile roles traditionally ascribed to them in Europe. The princess in the toybox, the doll dressed in yards of nylon tulle, floral corsage, diamanté necklace and tiara mirrors the changes that women were performing.

Barbie's Predecessors: the American Story

That the 1950s lady dolls were about self-confirmation and development through referencing the complex and elite code of high fashion is reiterated through the Barbie doll's alternate genealogy from the American fashion or glamour doll of the 1950s. The feminist elements that underpin Barbie's meanings, like much of the content of her extraordinary world of cross-reference, have an identifiable precursor. Such affirmation of female glamour as aspirational and liberative already emerged through the career of Madame Beatrice Alexander of New York, and informs the American side of Barbie's pedigree. Alexander is credited with presenting in 1955 the first successful fashion doll of the 1950s, Cissy – just over a century since Adelaide Huret introduced her fashion dolls in 1850. Alongside renditions of girls, toddlers and babies, from at least the 1930s onwards, Alexander always made realisations in doll form of singular women. These 'famous women' were deeply feminine and imbued with nostalgia and yet Alexander chose women who were seen in popular culture to exert a certain degree of de facto feminist agency or at least an agency of status.

The feminist power was expressed by Madame Alexander's production of Scarlett O'Hara dolls. Her first Scarlett dolls pre-dated the *Gone With the Wind* film, reaching the market in 1936, supported only by the already singular popularity of Margaret Mitchell's novel. Whilst subsequent models to the present day reproduced the well-known look of the film, the early Scarletts did not (Davis 2002: 22). They were Alexander's own visualisation of Scarlett in 1860s dress and wide picture hat, based on reading Mitchell's novel. That the book was regarded as racy adult literature, indeed the Catholic Church clearly identified it as morally disreputable (Taylor 1989: 36–7), would suggest that Alexander had a mature clientele in mind for her 'Scarletts'.

Gone With the Wind has been a potent site for the development of a de facto feminist consciousness among women who have often felt alienated from more academic feminist arenas (1989: 7–10, 52, 94, 101–105). Despite its racist and colonialist assumptions, as well as its arbitrary, slyly sensuous, stratagems of romance, the novel offered a vision of a world that was unique in popular culture from the 1930s to 1950s. It both soothed women's frustrations with their narrow options and experiences and also provided a rare validation of women's ability to manage challenge and responsibilities, offering like no other novel 'a world of omnipresent women and *intermittently* stable and dependable men' [my italics] (1989: 8). When asked by Helen Taylor, 'women described . . . their identification with and admiration of the strong and resourceful Scarlett, getting what she wants out of life – something many of them have obviously failed to do' (1989: 94). The novel had a particular resonance with women in Britain during the Second World War, and in Europe after the war, when it became widely known in many countries, as providing a metaphorical framework for processing memory and experience. *Gone With the Wind* especially validated the new responsibilities and the expectations and assumptions that women would uphold the good of the state and maintain 'business as usual' on the homefront through their own resources and initiatives. Therefore Alexander's Scarletts have affinity to Bild Lilli's tale of female perseverance and transcendence in the wake of wartime humiliation, thus indicating the parallel trajectories of Barbie's two genealogies.

However, Scarlett's potency as a symbolic figure is not only about surviving the Second World War and dealing with a crumbling and threatened social structure in which men frequently failed to live up to the position of power and privilege that the symbolic order ascribed to them. She still speaks to women who have few formal guidelines for the potential and placement of the feminine in the public world of power and commerce and the strategies that they must follow in order to survive. Helen Taylor suggests that there is even – in her own words – a 'Thatcher-ite' Scarlett for the 1980s and after. 'It is easy to imagine a modern dress version of GWTW with Scarlett doing very nicely on the Stock Exchange, comfortably ensconced in London's fashionable Docklands or New York's Upper East Side' (Taylor 1989: 101). Mary Rogers suggests that 'Barbie, Aunt Jemima and Scarlett O'Hara are fictive icons that let people imaginatively explore race, sexuality and femininity' (1999: 3).

Alexander also included *Little Women* dolls as perennial lines throughout her dollmaking career. Again the March girls have been potent female/feminist symbols in North American culture as well as much-loved figures from childhood reading. In various films down the generations the March girls have provided a lexicon of the possibilities and the values that North American women can exert at a given date: from the pre-Raphaelite saintly death of Meg; to the importance of a virtuous home in creating a backbone for a healthy nation; to the courage of women 'carrying-on' in war time whilst their men were defending the homeland; to the modern feminist remaking of Jo as independent, self-sufficient woman and aspiring professional, and finally heterosexual partner in a well-balanced marriage.

During the 1950s Queen Elizabeth II – an unlikely sister of the March girls and Scarlett O'Hara – was another staple line of the Alexander company. The Queen Elizabeth dolls indicate that Alexander had other motivations beyond developing merchandise from popular American culture. In a culture which begot the god-desses of Hollywood, who would necessarily need Queen Elizabeth II, especially as she is the direct descendant of the notorious and mad King George? Alexander was herself, as a New Yorker and daughter of an immigrant family that arrived in the United States in the late-nineteenth century, a quintessential North American child of the 'melting pot'. Her dolls were made in New York as a logical extension of the ragtrade which had provided employment to so many immigrants. She came from a family of Russian-Jewish descent whose departure from Europe was believed to have been provoked by Czarist anti-Semitism. A family legend claims that Alexander's father and siblings were killed in a pogrom, with only her preg-nant mother and the yet unborn Bertha (who later renamed herself as the more aristocratic Beatrice) left alive to emigrate to America. Other family members outline a less emotively dramatic history of migration, suggesting that her father was not slain by Cossacks, but died in New York when Beatrice was an infant.[8] Her family history makes a familial tradition of monarchical support even less likely.

In comparison to Alexander, one would expect British dollmakers, from Augusta Montanari in the 1850s to Peggy Nisbet in the 1960s and 1970s, to directly express their affection for the British Royal Family in an astutely business-like fashion by marketing royal portraits. In turn monarchist sentiments amongst English doll buyers down the generations have provided a secure consumer base for various British 'royal' dolls, from the wax infants representing Queen Victoria's children, to bisque dolls designed for the British trade, such as the German Schoenau and Hoffmeister *Prinzess Elizabeth* doll of the early-1930s, to Nisbet's hard plastic dolls representing a cavalcade of royal personalities, past and present.

Even in the 1930s Alexander had produced royal princess dolls as a natural extension to her other celebrity children, the Dionnes. These American-made doll princesses already assimilated Elizabeth and Margaret into popular culture, long before British tabloid newspapers moved from saccharine hagiography to prying sensationalism in their treatment of 'the Royals', or long before Diana had danced with John Travolta. The de facto North American peers of the 'little princesses' were not only the Dionne Quintuplets, but also other dolls representing high-profile children of the 1930s such as Ideal's Shirley Temple, Judy Garland and Deanna Durbin. Other royal-type dolls were produced by Alexander in the 1950s, again showing her affection for all things British and royal. They include her Grenadier Guards, who have the strange gender ambiguity of all of Alexander's surrealist, androgynous males. Such males range from David the Rabbi, to Union and Confederate Officers to Harley Davidson Riders (albeit dashing and more socially acceptable leather-clad 1920s motorcycle riders, not present-day socially marginalised 'bikies' or the urban, salaried, upper middle-class professional wannabes, referenced by Mattel's Harley Davidson Barbie and Ken). Alexander's males all share a strange inter-gender characterisation, due to the use of standard female faces with the wide-eyed vulnerable looks seen throughout all Madame Alexander dolls. The star of her males was a golden-blonde Prince Philip doll from 1953. In dress naval uniform and cape Philip could easily be mistaken for a portrait doll of Liberace, but he was an appropriate consort for Madame's glamorous queens.

It is the irrationality of Alexander's dedication to Queen Elizabeth II as a fixture in her annual doll line alongside the Scarletts, the March Sisters and the ballerinas during the 1950s that identifies the feminist potential in the Queen as a guiding and inspirational figure. Glenn Mandeville suggests that in 1953 Alexander, like many North Americans, had found the televised coronation fascinating (2001a: 52). Whilst Alexander's first set of coronation dolls was a promotional commission from a Brooklyn department store, Abraham and Strauss, the decade-long reap-pearance of the British monarch, in an impossibly youthful and glamorous incarna-tion and differing evening gowns and regalia each year, reflected Madame's own taste. It took two decades for Alexander to contemplate issuing an equally impos-sible and glamorous rendition of the American First Ladies released sequentially throughout the mid-1970s. Her interpretation of the Presidents' wives as romantic beauties gilded the lily of their generally obscure status,[9] even amongst the North American public; whereas Queen Elizabeth, Scarlett, Jo and her sisters (and also the ballerinas if they were read as Margot Fonteyn and the Royal Ballet) were all exalted and paradigmatic figures of wish-fulfilment. The Queen Elizabeths

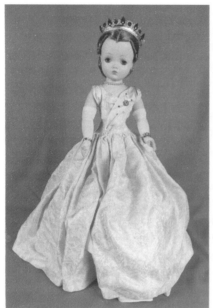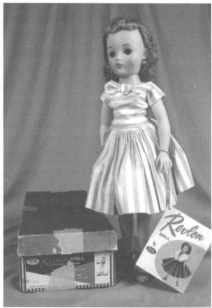

Figure 6.2 Left to right: Queen Elizabeth II in original dress by Madame Alexander 1950s; Miss Revlon in original dress by Ideal 1956 or later, image by courtesy of McMasters Harris Auctions, USA.

disappeared from the annual doll issues after the early 1960s. However in 2002 the Alexander company issued two new portraits of the Queen, not reflecting her current age and image but as a young woman in a white New Look evening dress and miniature versions of the British Robes of State. Every year the Alexander company issues a new set of March sisters and several Scarletts. Whilst Scarlett always appears, her retinue of characters from the book, film and the Civil War era generally change from year to year.

Alexander had passionate convictions about the characters and identities of her dolls. They reflected the Jewish immigrants' respect for self-improvement and education. In particular they enact her clear memories of 'escaping' her childhood in New York's East Side through reading and day dreaming. Fashion and appearances in turn-of-the-century New York were a stimulus for the young Beatrice to better herself as well as an indication of class differences.

> 'When I was 11 or 12,' she remembered, 'I realized that there were poor people and there were rich people, and I leaned towards the rich. I wanted to have a carriage and a hat with ostrich feathers.' Hannah [her mother] assumed her daughter would achieve these goals by 'marry[ing] well' and joked that it would take three husbands to support Beatrice in the manner she desired. (Jewish Women's Archive Project 2001c)

Thus too Alexander saw no inconsistencies between her mission to create dolls who represented 'substance' and power for women and in her presentation to the public of a doll wearing high-style fashions. She defended the uplifting purpose of her Cissy doll, even in the face of resistance from WASP American society. She stated that she held Cissy back from the marketplace for several years because the Daughters of the American Revolution would disapprove (Jewish Women's Archive Project 2001d). Barbie was similarly delayed for the reason of her supposedly inappropriate eroticism. Having decided to launch the doll in 1955, Alexander did not waver in her belief in Cissy even when buyers at the New York Toy Show regarded her as a male novelty for the stag party and bachelor trade, again prefiguring the unease that Barbie would occasion amongst wholesale buyers in 1959. Alexander insisted that Cissy be presented in her nylons and elegant underwear. This was not an erotic gesture, but just provided the appropriate underpinnings to a spreading New Look dress. In Alexander's opinion Cissy did not force adult sexuality upon girls, rather she gave little girls access to high fashion. Cissy was advertised as a 'child's' dream come true' (Carrillo 1999: 62). As in nineteenth-century France, dolls were frequently shipped in the 1950s wearing underwear or intimate garments.

Alexander also did not regard Cissy, the high fashion model, as incongruous amongst her carefully researched 'heroines' of ballet, opera and literature and 'great women of history'. Such dolls were staples of the Alexander company as well as the more expected dollmaking fare of babies, children, nursery rhyme and fairy tale characters. The beautiful luxury fashion doll Cissy could be likened to Queen Elizabeth II or the perennial classical ballerinas, including one in particular, the Margot Ballerina of 1954, whom collectors believe to be a specific tribute to Margot Fonteyn, as 'a flawless performer of pristine reserve' (Sargent 1997: 46) and inspirational to girls. Cissy differed only in that her 'divine right' to rule was the authority of the Parisian couture house rather than the British constitutional monarchy or the discipline of professional ballet training. Due to her popularity, Cissy stayed in production for seven years until 1962. By this date the larger fashion dolls were no longer able to maintain viable sales against Barbie. When Cissy was launched, Alexander had already been publicly commended in North America for her fashion design ability. The clothes worn by dolls made by the Alexander company won the American Fashion Academy Award for three consecutive years during the early-1950s, in open competition with manufacturers of adult apparel. Glenn Mandeville suggests that the choice of a dollmaker above actual garment manufacturers was controversial, 'for three years in a row, she won the prestigious "Fashion Academy Award" which on the surface sounds like no big deal, but the facts are that the contest is open to *all* designers of clothing for real people – Madame Alexander had won this award for doll-sized fashions! Many in the fashion industry simply could not believe it' (2001b). As a dollmaker,

Alexander's winning an award intended for the mainstream garment trade can also indicate the breadth of her cultural ambition in relation to dolls. In the early 1960s, at the time when Mattel's dolls were overtaking Alexander's in the toymarket, she moved into the apparel business, until her husband warned about 'too many orders, spreading you too thin' (McWhorter 2003: 64).

Cissy's impact upon her original audience is outlined by a North American doll collector writing in response to a millennial quest to identify the 'doll of the century':

> My favorite doll would have to be the 1950s Madame Alexander Cissy dolls. To me they represent the high-fashion fantasy that every little girl once dreamed of emulating. With their couture dresses inspired by Dior and many other famous clothing designers of the era, they bring out the hidden glamour gal in every woman. From their lovely shoes to their fancy hats, Cissy dolls will always represent to me the ultimate combination of wearable art and casual elegance. (Lucas 2000: 58)

Diana Lucas's account indicates Cissy's contribution to popular understanding of gender and fashion. The recollections of 1950s childhoods, quoted at the start of this chapter, indicate the almost magical power of 'the Dress' in female imaginations and the ubiquitous, concomitant dreams of female transcendence through 'beauty, high fashion and the right man' (Caviale 1997: 37; Spunner 1999: 14). Cissy brought all these elements directly into the play time of her young owners, even before they could discover the cinema and the instructions and advice on life patterns that it presented. Another millennial countdown of dolls also included Cissy as eighth out of twelve on an internet list of the 'Dolls of the Century':

> Madame Alexander's Cissy is the adult-shaped, high heeled glamorous fashion doll that paved the way for modern fashion dolls as we know them! Without Cissy which was first sold in 1955, Barbie, Miss Revlon, Tammy and all of the other fashion dolls, which have followed might not have been. Cissy was considered quite scandalous in her time. (van Patten 2000)

Cissy's wardrobe was noted for its luxury fabrics and trims of the highest quality. Some of her dresses were in real silk and the scaling of printed motifs to the doll showed much felicity. Likewise the millinery paired to the outfits not only featured a wide variety of current styles but again was distinguished by the quality of materials used and the perfect understanding of the potential of scale and technique, drawing upon all the expected elements of the era such as artificial flowers, veiling and fine straws, but in small scale. Cissy's wardrobe captured the extremely romantic approach to millinery of the early and mid-1950s. Dior was as influential in setting the directions in 1950s millinery as he was in other areas of fashion. He was always concerned that hats presented the perfect complement to his garments (Genty 1994: 21). The components of Cissy's dresses and accessories were matched in quality by the thoroughness and intelligence of the interpretation of contemporary fashion. Within the parameters of updated technology and production methods, the range and detail of Cissy's clothing and its precise replication of current styles and its evocation of upper-class lifestyles resembles that of the Parisienne of a century earlier.

> Madame Alexander used all the skill, creativeness, and resources of her company in producing a wardrobe for her diminutive debutante. Cissy was available as a dressed doll in everything from basic lingerie to ball gowns. Madame Alexander designed numerous costumes for Cissy that featured daring décolletage, dropped waists and full sweeping skirts. A complete wardrobe was also available separately and included lingerie, casual attire, sports wear, evening clothes, shoes, hosiery and millinery. The right outfit and accessories were available to act out in fantasy every aspect of a young debutante's life. (Carrillo 1999: 62)

There is a repeated motif in various discussions of Cissy in that, concurrent to emphasising the class and status of the doll, her potentially transgressive sexuality is referenced in order to demonstrate not her tawdriness, as generally emerges from discussions around Barbie, but to demonstrate her avant-garde and innovative status. Her décolleté dresses are singled out by Joseph Carrillo; Denise van Patten notes that Cissy was considered scandalous (van Patten 2000) and Alexander herself seems almost proud that the Daughters of the American Revolution (presumably defined as conservative Anglo-Saxon Protestants) may have found her doll too forward (Jewish Women's Archive Project 2001d). Yet all these recent accounts concurrently emphasise Cissy as a symbol of quality. If Cissy challenges expected morality and the limited options surrounding dolls, her superiority is located in a 'progressive' outlook. Thus Cissy follows the classic trajectory of the avant-garde, which outrages the bourgeois norm and acquires status as avatar or innovation. Possibly this suspension of moral judgement indicates Cissy's kinship with high fashion, which in recent years frequently explicitly references sexuality, yet vox populi extends a relative degree of tolerance and elasticity towards high fashion's sexual content. This elastic indulgence only breaks briefly at certain extremes such as 'heroin chic' or extremely anorexic or juvenile models in parades or photoshoots, but it is soon restored.

If we assign responsibility for the reappearance of the fashion doll in the North American dollmarket in the mid-1950s to Beatrice Alexander, it again indicates that certain major strategic shifts in the outlook of dollmaking companies and the culture of producing and purchasing dolls were made by women. Augusta Montanari and Adelaide Huret overturned the limited range of possibilities in the doll marketplace. As said earlier, Huret developed ideas around the practical commodification of style that pre-dated the emergence of the House of Worth. In marketing and reifying the elusive ethos of class and glamour in a modern society as an object that could be freely traded, Huret was able to coalesce what were hitherto invisible ideas about reputation and style and materialise them around the object of the fashion doll. She turned reputation into something that could be freely traded as a commodity. The German doll reform was led by women, such as Marion Kaulitz with the Munich Art Dolls and Käthe Kruse with her cloth dolls. Barbie's success was fostered by the vision of Ruth Handler, and, as I have said, the Barbie doll could be regarded as a creative production that has an unusually wide distribution for a woman's artwork (Peers 1996: 6), especially in that misogynist strain of post-Enlightenment modernism that denies women the capacity for original thought.

Alexander dolls were regarded as the highest quality in American doll production in the 1950s, and the direction that Beatrice Alexander set with Cissy was closely followed by other companies. Among the best known of her compatriots were Ideal's Miss Revlon, American Character Doll Corporation's Sweet Sue Sophisticate, Vogue Doll Company's Jill, Horsman's Cindy, and The Coty Girl, marketed by Aranbee. The Coty Girl resembled similar products especially Miss Revlon (Mandeville 2000: 74–5), but the Coty Girl had an advantage in the teeming marketplace through direct association with a Paris-based company, albeit in cosmetics rather than in a fashion house such as the Schiaparelli, Effanbee and Virga dolls. The Coty Girl's wardrobe substantially emphasised her Parisian identity. Her black asymmetrical picture hat is a particularly dramatic example of the 1950s styling for dolls and was also used as her logo. The packaging graphics were intended to coordinate with the known styling of the cosmetic company. As with the Schiaparelli Virga collaboration, North American toy companies' desire to brand their products with the already famous names from Paris indicates the permeation of Haute Couture into daily life and values in North America. Yet customer recognition of these European names was somewhat limited, as the most successful dolls were not the Schiaparelli or Coty tie-ins, but local products that emulated or glossed French style yet were firmly based in the North American marketplace: Alexander's Cissy and Ideal's Miss Revlon. Within a year of her launch, the Coty Girl had a square dance dress in her wardrobe indicating the importance of North American as much as Parisian values to families buying dolls.

By the late-1950s every doll company in North America produced a glamorous lady amongst their range. There were many cheaper copies and dolls from smaller American companies. Fashionable lady dolls appeared in supermarkets and neighbourhood grocery stores. Even these cheap versions were sold in packaging that indicated their status as glamorous models or upper-class belles, in small towns as well as large, across the United States. The cultural importance of these mature lady dolls in American constructions of fashion and style in the 1950s was acknowledged by a relatively rare presentation of 1950s dolls in a public gallery context. In 2000, the Mint Museum of Art in Charlotte, North Carolina, presented a survey of vintage bridal dolls, as an adjunct to an exhibition *To Have and to Hold: 135 Years of Bridal Fashion*. The text for the exhibition describes the 1950s as a 'golden age' for 'high fashion dolls and doll clothing that mirrored top styles by European and American designers . . . In the early-1950s fashion dolls were again popular as female dolls displayed adult features and arched heel shoes' (Mint Museum of Art 2001).

It was not only the haunting power of fashion as key icon in the 1950s that encouraged the development of these fashion dolls, or the fact that these dolls captured public fascination with high fashion. Post-Second World War America was an insatiable marketplace for new ideas and products. Plastic fashion dolls were but one of a myriad of products that satisfied that unceasing demand for diversity and novelty, if not luxury, in the marketplace. Fashion dolls of the 1950s belonged to an unparalleled expansion of doll and toy manufacturing and retailing in postwar North America. Large-scale companies such as Jumeau and Märklin had earlier understood, and developed, the potential of the toy trade in a modern industrial society, but such companies had co-existed with many home-based workshops and small production units. Only the 1950s brought the thorough assimilation of the child's play world into an integrated industrial marketplace. Generally this editing and containment of the supposedly 'free' world of the child, especially by North American toy companies and large industry, has alarmed cultural critics over the past four decades (Rundle 2001: 1, 4). Companies such as Mattel, Ideal and Hasbro were at the forefront of this development. As noted in relation to the French bébé, the myth of the 'innocent' child could be read as a flattering self-mirror of the supposedly free and self-determined world of the Enlightenment thinker; so the child whose 'childhood' is hijacked by Coca Cola or other corporations becomes a metaphor, in the mind of some observers, for the lack of freedom that is the reality for the supposedly 'free' post-capitalist citizen. Thus, for some, not only does the Barbie doll represent the personification of the malign influence of capitalism, but she genders that malign influence explicitly female. 'Mattel promotes capitalism and the unequal distribution of resources by glamorising a character with a huge amount of apparently unearned disposable cash and . . . a disproportionate amount of luxury items' (Rand 1995: 8). 'The cold war has been won and Barbie appears to have been one of the generals – or perhaps a major weapon' (Varney 2002: 43).

The plethora of toys designed, marketed and sold in North America indicated that its middle-class citizens enjoyed a material prosperity without historical precedent. The development and cultivation of this range of consumer choice became the hallmark of the postwar era. The multiplicity of new dolls in the 1950s was a natural result of the expanding market and could be regarded as just one of many new products from cars to fast foods that personify the burgeoning consumerism of this era. Yet the doll – especially the Barbie doll – also became an ideal forum in which to take stock and document the visual patterns and material culture of this changing postwar society. Glenn Mandeville quotes *Life* magazine in 1954 regarding the new prominence of toys in prosperous postwar America: 'Never before so much for so few'. Mandeville adds 'These children were pampered as no other generation before them had been. Their toys would soon be a reflection of that attitude' (2001b). The sheer numbers of dolls and toys and the changing of the most popular materials for dollmaking from porcelain, wood and composition to plastic also represented the man-made substance and consumer revolution in North America during the 1950s. The difference between the French bisque and the American plastic dolls was the expansion of the middle-class domestic marketplace. Yet, as said above, one could also argue that from amongst the multitude of 'must-have' toys that denoted prosperous family life in North America the doll, like high fashion, represented a particularly significant cultural expression in the 1950s. Bild Lilli further ratifies the special position that dolls play in 1950s social history.

Barbie herself emerged from this postwar expansion of the toy trade. Mattel's development of the Barbie line in some ways was an adroit and alert refocussing of the often large and elaborate dolls of the mid- to late-1950s. The fashionable lady dolls of the 1950s were – despite the plastic moulded bodies and stilettos or the yards of nylon tulle as signs of technology – not too far removed from nineteenth-century Parisian dollmaking ateliers in conception. Barbie moved the fashion doll into a format that could be unequivocally assimilated into late-twentieth-century habits and lifestyles. The success with which Ruth Handler and Mattel madeover the 1950s glamour doll ensured that modern plastic fashion dolls would live long beyond the demise of crinoline petticoats with net underlays and rope inserts as a fashion item, or the fascination with the formality of postwar French fashion that these larger dolls expressed. Barbie was small, compact and comfortably held in the hand. A daytime walk through any shopping mall in a 'Western' based culture will reveal parents accompanied by children who are firmly clutching Barbies or 'knock-off' or 'clone' Barbies in various stages of disorder in dress and hairstyle. The larger fashion dolls, who were produced earlier in the 1950s – say of twenty inches or more – could not be comfortably carried about with such casualness.

Barbie's small size means that acquiring and storing more than one example of the doll and her extended entourage of family and friends became relatively easy. Multiple holdings of dolls – since the 1970s many child owners have more than one Barbie as well as 'friends and family' – of course mean more sales of clothing. Barbie's wardrobe integrated the homely with the elegant, so she could be both a model from Paris and the girl next door; it was thus ensured that all tastes found something appealing about the doll. What set Barbie apart and established her as a relatively new and unfamiliar format in dollmaking was duplicated from Lilli. Through Lilli's compact format, Barbie provided an effective model for presenting fashion on a smaller scale than the substantial glamour dolls, who, like the bébé, could be quite large, even up to three feet in size. Lilli proved that an eleven-and-a-half inch reduction could be popular. Her slimness and elongation gave the illusion of greater height. The slimness and poise implied particularly by Lilli's design, high-heeled and shapely legged with poised fingers, also cross-referenced paper dolls of the 1940s. Due to referencing a foreign doll as prototype, Barbie could not be dismissed as simply a reduced version of existing dolls, as could the small-sized Little Miss Revlon or Cissette. Barbie's foreign source made her a novelty in the oversupplied United States fashion doll market.

Mattel also realigned the 1950s fashion doll to ensure that she was effective in her appearance and persona, yet could be produced economically and in large quantities. Barbie was always intended to be produced in higher volume and to serve a wider market than the Alexander dolls, akin to the broad audience for Ideal dolls. The reduction of scale meant that some detail and elaboration could be removed from the dresses without there being any overall perceivable loss of the impact of the fashionable replication. Careful sampling and product development ensured that fabrics which performed appropriately within the constraints of scale and cost were specified. Designer Carole Spencer recalls how she had to work with a 'textile expert testing many fabrics' in the 1960s. 'We did not have all the right fabrics and trying to find the right quality we did not have the right finishes. The things that you can do today are amazing with the fabrics that will accept all this. We just did not have the technology that exists today' (Westenhouser 1994: 41). Barbie's famous tiny waist, so often denounced as unhealthy and unnatural, is moulded small so that there will not be a build-up of fabrics around her waist when she is fully dressed. 'She is one sixth the size of a person, but her fabrics are suited for people. Barbie's middle . . . had to be disproportionately narrow to look proportional in clothes. The intersection of a waistband of a skirt involves four layers of cloth' (Lord 1994: 12–13). Even the finest fabrics are much larger in proportion to the doll than they are on a human scale and their potential for drape is therefore more limited in designing for dolls. With the expansion of the adult collector dollmarket, the limitations of the Barbie size for construction and design are also becoming more apparent – as opposed to the fifteen inch Gene to eighteen inch Huret size range. These larger dolls are again finding favour for their increased scale, which facilitates a greater range of both materials and construction techniques, especially as regards accessorising and trimming outfits.

Until the arrival of Barbie, Ideal's Miss Revlon was perhaps the most widely distributed fashion doll in North America. Ideal is among the most successful mid-twentieth-century American doll firms. Denise van Patten describes Ideal as 'THE [sic] play dolls for generations of little girls – Shirley, Betsey Wetsey, Toni, Mary Hartlin, Betsy McCall, Saucy Walker, Miss Revlon, Tammy and Chrissy' (2000). Ideal were propelled to this level by their best-selling composition dolls of the

1930s, which were 'celebrity' dolls and beyond the scope of this text. It is enough to state that dolls such as the Shirley Temple doll ensured that the market for American dolls or American-designed dolls would not fail during the 1930s, as little girls internationally demanded a 'Shirley'. Other popular Ideal dolls of the era were portraits of celebrities, equally desirable to little girls, including Judy Garland, Deanna Durbin and Sonja Heine. Likewise the finances of the Alexander doll company were underpinned during the same era by another best-seller, the Dionne Quintuplets. The girls were shown at various stages of their lives in doll form. The Dionnes were a dollmaker's dream in that every dress, every accessory, needed to be replicated fivefold, even if the 'sets' of Dionnes consist of five identical dolls differentiated by the names embroidered on their dresses and the colour-coding of each garment. Beyond the official licensed Alexander Dionnes, throughout the 1930s many dollmakers and toy companies, including those in Japan, sold dolls in groups of five as 'Quints'. Even if the name 'Dionne' was not used, buyers and children knew that dolls sold in sets of five represented the celebrity sisters.

Ideal have been described as 'not always the first to implement an idea, but Ideal dolls were always good quality and available at an affordable price' (van Patten 2000). Ideal demonstrated how rival doll companies immediately adapted Alexander's Cissy. Miss Revlon, who appeared in 1956, was more reasonably priced than Cissy. A fully dressed Miss Revlon cost about half the price of a Cissy in her notorious underwear. Sales rocketed and within a year more Miss Revlons were being sold in the United States than any other doll. Glenn Mandeville cites *Playthings*, the North American toy trade equivalent of *Women's Wear Daily* as marketplace bible, which listed Miss Revlon as the top-selling doll for 1956 in the United States (2001d: 54). This indicates not only the importance of lower price in gaining a wide audience but also the level of popularity enjoyed by fashion dolls in the mid- to late-1950s, even before Barbie was launched in 1959.

Miss Revlon's packaging indicated how the correct presentation of a fashionable appearance became itself the very definition of a woman. A list of fashion accessories textually constructed a complete and mature woman:

> Little girls whisper . . . 'Now I have a BIG sister!'
> The beautiful, beautiful Revlon Doll by Ideal
> A teen age sister with
> A real girl's figure
> High heels
> Sheer nylon stockings
> High fashion clothes
> Elegant jewellery
> So beautiful her name just had to be Revlon.

> (Anon c.late 1950s)

A sketch of the doll in full, twirling skirts in a dancing pose accompanied this blank verse tribute to fashion. Miss Revlon's wardrobe is particularly noteworthy. It is made from homely enough fabrics with comfortable references to homespun, pioneering American values: stripes and ginghams, clean fresh cottons, but cut and sewn with an effective sense of visual rhythms and a 'smart' appearance.

Around the late-1950s there was a craze for miniature fashion dolls. These dolls would rapidly disappear from the shops following the success of Barbie. Again Madame Alexander was at the forefront of the new development, with a small doll called Cissette, followed in turn by a ten-and-a-half inch, 'Little Miss Revlon'. To compete against Cissette, Ideal first marketed a ten-and-a-half inch doll called the Crown Princess in 1957. Her name reflected the fascination with royalty that ensured that Madame Alexander's annual Queen Elizabeths found many North American homes. Despite her regal name, the Crown Princess was quite a cheap doll and the next year, 1958, Ideal issued Little Miss Revlon, a more expensive doll of greater quality and solidity in her materials and more flexible in her joints (Mandeville 2001d: 56). The Crown Princess's special novelty was that she was supplied with a pearlised plastic tiara, indicating her rank. Her clothes were mostly in cotton and not as elaborate as those of Cissy or Sweet Sue Sophisticate. Judith Izen collected oral history accounts from former Ideal employees who suggested that Ideal's chief dress designer, Mary Brauer, found working on the ten-and-a-half inch scale irksome. In comparison to larger fashion dolls by Ideal, therefore, these small dolls, the Crown Princess and Little Miss Revlon, were provided with clothing that 'lack[ed] . . . special pizzazz' (Izen 2001: 102). Still, most of the dresses for the small Ideal dolls were variations on the New Look silhouette in various materials, especially printed cottons but also in some more glamorous fabrics, such as an iridescent checked taffeta bias-cut skirt worn with a red satin fez and a bolero jacket. There were long evening dresses in sparkling lace and other glittering fabrics, coats with faux leopard trim and oriental cheongsam detailings in a brocade lounging outfit, overall a cross section of fashionable themes and trends of the mid- to late-1950s. Little Miss Revlon could not compete with Barbie and was discontinued in 1960.

Another iconic adult doll of the 1950s was Jill, by Vogue. The Vogue Doll Company was first founded as a doll dressmaking company with fashions designed by Jennie Adler Graves. Like Alexander, Graves built up a substantial commercial enterprise through dolls. She started dressing dolls for friends and family in the 1920s,[10] but her designs proved to be so popular that she opened the Vogue Doll Shoppe in 1922, dressing high-quality imported German bisque dolls made by Armand Marseille, and Kammer and Reinhardt; they were mostly little girl dolls wearing children's clothes, including the novelty mascot *Just Me* doll by Marseille. The *Just Me* doll was particularly associated with Graves' name in North America, more than that of its German manufacturer. In the 1930s Graves was selling imported dolls to retailers across the country. These imported dolls wore clothes she designed and had manufactured under her supervision in North America. By the late-1940s, with the loss of dolls from German suppliers during the war, she was commissioning American production of exclusive dolls in composition then later in hard plastic (Ledbetter 2001; Vogue Doll Company 2002). Her most popular doll was Ginny, a little girl doll. M.G. Lord memorably described poor Ginny as 'pot bellied, pugnosed, flat chested' (1994: 40).

Most of Graves' dolls did not engage with high fashion, but in 1959 Graves entered the fashion doll stakes with an elegant beauty with breasts, feet moulded for high heels and polish on her finger and toenails – all signs of a doll's mature persona in the 1950s – named Jill, sold as Ginny's 'Big Sister'. Not only did Jill allow Vogue Dolls to enter new fields without changing and undermining the image of their proven, successful child dolls, but she also acclimatised the elegance of Haute Couture to the American home. Jill was marketed with the slogan 'the elegance and grace of sophistication, charm and exquisite styles' (Izen 1998: 15), a mantra of aspirational, escapist glamour that immediately indicates how far Dior penetrated the domestic sphere or even the juvenile market. Through the 'big sister' identity, a solution that Vogue was the first to devise, the very different and ladylike Jill could be as directly accessible as Ginny without the latter losing any of her cute, well-loved and unpretentiously approachable identity. Ironically Jill's wardrobe was designed by the real 'Ginny', Virginia Graves Carlson, Jenny Graves' daughter and the popular doll's namesake. Jill is also notable because long before Ken arrived on the scene, she was given a boyfriend named Geoff, allowing Jill to take part in the courtship rituals so important in the 1950s. Jill was among the most widely recognised of the fashion dolls of the 1950s. Glenn Mandeville suggests that she particularly represented the growing profile of North American teenage subcultures in the late 1950s (2001c). The Jill and Geoff personae indicated that the new teenage lifestyles and especially dating and courtship rituals were beginning to acquire centrality as points of cultural reference and indications of 'normality', despite – and simultaneous with – anxieties about teenage delinquency and promiscuity becoming a focus of greater public discussion.

Jill's teenage persona was a suitable interlocutor between Paris and middle America. Whilst Cissy was sold in bra, panties and nylons, Jill arrived in her new home wearing a black nylon leotard, with a scarf-sarong, slightly avant-garde and beatnik but not quite as risqué as underwear. This morphing between the distant and the familiar would be seen in the Barbie wardrobe. American popular culture was represented by a 'Western' rodeo outfit and a circular rock and roll skirt in printed felt featuring musical and rock motifs. Such novelty skirts have become a cliché of popular pastiches and recapitulations of 1950s fashion, in fancy dress and amateur theatre, but Jill indicates their currency in middle-market fashion, as understood at the time. The rock and roll skirt is again an instance of dolls documenting the vernacular practices of fashion. Other garments worn by Jill present a more matronly interpretation of 1950s modes. They include a sensible, but crisply tailored, lemon taffeta New Look dress, with a high neckline but a very wide skirt, which suggests both a certain neat sobriety as well as the formal chic that was the expected public presentation of the feminine; and a red evening dress with a hailspot net underskirt visible beneath the skirt and a more showy ballerina-length cocktail dress in net over satin, with floral corsage and ribbon appliqué on the net. Her upmarket accessories included a white rabbit stole, pearl earrings, a charm bracelet, rhinestone-trimmed sandals and various hats, fascinators, veils and snoods in velvet and net to match different garments. The veiled hats in particular lent an air of sophistication. Jill barely survived the launch of Barbie by two years and was withdrawn in 1961.

Sweet Sue Sophisticate, by the American Character Doll Corporation, was another high-profile glamorous doll of the 1950s. She came in a number of sizes, and was particularly notable for the beauty of her formalwear, such as the fuchsia tulle and black velvet ensemble discussed above. Another elaborately draped evening dress was in ruched pale blue tulle. Many of her garments feature miniature bouffant petticoats to create the full crinoline effect. When in pristine condition, the dresses deploy the possibilities of tulles, nets and organzas as overlays and trims to the fullest extent. These garments were available in various versions to match the sizes of the dolls. Sweet Sue Sophisticate came in a number of variations on the same basic doll; all were manufactured by the American Character Doll Corporation. The doll named 'Sweet Sue', without the appellation 'Sophisticate', was as Midge was to Barbie: a less dramatic doll who could appeal to those buyers who found the key doll unacceptable. Sweet Sue Sophisticate was also marketed as the second version of the Toni doll and sold under the name of American Beauty. Ironically, despite her name, the American Beauty is European in her style orientation. Glenn Mandeville writes that the madeover Toni doll was 'a high heeled vixen with adult features.'

> Deluxe and rare models had flirty eyes that glanced from side to side that some called provocative. The outfits were very sophisticated and spoke of women that were enjoying themselves being just that. No male partners or babies were part of the play value to these dolls. It was all about growing up and having fun. Times were changing quickly. (Mandeville 2001c)

Other commentators respond to her escapist, exceptional quality. A collector writing on her homepages has no doubt about Sweet Sue's identity: 'Queen of the dolls. So enchanting that she looks like a movie star' (Kruger 2002).

To describe Sweet Sue Sophisticate as a film star immediately defines her beauty in relation to established cultural canons. The identity 'film star' expresses a certain over-the-top, but measurable, perfection of beauty. 'Film star' also suggests material wealth and exemption from behavioural codes that confine the middle class and untalented. It also expresses certain quintessential American dreams of cruising forth to transcendence. The Gene Marshall doll is seen to express these same values, even to the point of being an autobiographical symbol of her creator (Anon 2001: 8; Sarasohn-Kahn 2001a). Above all to name a woman/ doll as a 'film star' is to cast her as an icon, camp and peerless. Only perhaps in her name did Sweet Sue Sophisticate achieve less than perfection. 'Sweet' seems too bland an adjective to attach to this compelling mannequin and Sue seemed too plain and everyday a name for her.

Some lady dolls directly inspired by American dolls were also marketed in the 1950s by British doll companies. These dolls are much rarer than their North American counterparts as fewer were made. Examples of stylish dolls, dressed with much care and attention as Cissy or Sweet Sue Sophisticate, can be identified from such major plastic doll manufacturers as Pedigree, Rosebud and Chiltern. Chiltern was a superior quality firm amongst British post-1945 dollmakers. The range of British dollmakers' responses to the North American fashion doll is only beginning to be explored. A doll found in a Melbourne antique shop in 2001 indicates that Pedigree sent moulds for adult female dolls to one of its subsidiary factories in the British Commonwealth – in this case Australia. The doll was a clear copy of the Cissy/Miss Revlon genre.[11] Pedigree launched a number of fashion dolls sold under various names, including the 1950s Pin-Up doll – a British home perm doll, Little Miss Vogue, in 1961, and earlier during the 1950s Elizabeth, denoting the Queen's iconic status as exemplar of English womanhood. Elizabeth was sold through *Woman* magazine with a wardrobe designed by the magazine's resident 'fashion expert' Veronica Scott (Mansell 1995: 7–8). The doll dressed by major British designers c.1954, Virginia, also referenced the British monarchy. Her name prompted memories of Queen Elizabeth I, but her up-to-date fashion invoked the 'new' Elizabeth and the 'new' Elizabethan era that was such a catchcry around the time of the 'Festival of Britain' and the early years of the Queen's reign.

An account of the Miss Revlon doll by a present-day collector indicates how these glamour dolls introduced 1950s dress codes to young girls:

> Little girls feeling very grown up and into makeup decided to add glamour time to their play time. Her adult figure and high heeled feet matched perfectly to an adult style wardrobe . . . She wore stockings, in which the seams were always perfectly straight. Miss Revlon had pierced ears for her pearl earrings. Her makeup was very adult and flawless. She had rooted saran hair that had a bright sheen and little girls loved to wash and style the hair. (Davis 2001)

The repetition of the term 'perfect' in relation to the self-presentation of Miss Revlon's straight-seamed stockings and her ability to match 'an adult style wardrobe' indicates not only the values of public self-presentation that were expected from all women, but also the instructive directions of Miss Revlon's glamour. The taxonomy of Miss Revlon's successful mastery of the codes of beauty indicates the particular locations of well-known signs denoting female responsibility and self-management: straight stockings, high heels, clean hair with a 'bright sheen', cosmetics, a maturely styled wardrobe. Yet as the article indicates, this rule was not only coercive; it denoted material well-being as her earrings were made of 'pearls'. At all points Miss Revlon indicated 'maturity' and adult responsibility in her beauty. In her perfection she promised a deliverance from the abjectivity and dependence of the child state. Miss Revlon's beauty was not sybaritic: it denoted that little girls who played with Miss Revlon felt 'very grown up' to engage with her 'adult' styles of dress and make-up, and even pierced ears. The latter suggested that the rituals of beauty actually interacted with and altered the body's physicality and naturalness.

Miss Revlon indicated that empowerment could be achieved by a young girl aspiring to full adulthood through dress and self-presentation codes. This access to self-management again suggests that the glamour of the 1950s carried elements of feminism as well as oppression. In regard to the centrality of the feminine as a cultural metaphor, this glamour of self-presentation was not only a responsibility for women to carry, but it also indicated their enigmatic power in the symbolic hierarchy. Small, strange and generally overlooked, the dolls of the 1950s may still be relatively invisible in cultural overviews of the period, but from Bild Lilli through Cissy to Miss Revlon they reference the feminine as a state that is not closed. They engage in the double speak of empowerment as much as oppression.

–7–

Not Only a Pretty Face: Towards the New Millennium with the Designer Doll

There is nothing more boring than a really beautiful person who has nothing to say. Have you ever sat next to someone who is really good looking but incredibly vapid?

Gwynneth Paltrow qtd in *MX* (2002: 23)

The preceding narratives of dollmaking have indicated how couture and dollmaking, once conjoined in France at c.1855 had separated by 1900. Dollmaking likewise was separated from much mainstream Anglo-European cultural activity throughout the twentieth century. Exchange only happened in exceptional circumstances, in the shadow of extreme political and military threats to French sovereignty and identity. However beyond the academy and the fine arts, popular enthusiasm for French Haute Couture and the assimilation of Haute Couture into vernacular female experience produced a de facto union between French style and the burgeoning American toy trade.

French couture influences on North American dollmaking found a congenial base in a rapidly expanding doll marketplace buoyed up by advances in man-made materials technology and a sense of domestic plenitude amongst makers and consumers alike. Marketing's proactive generation of discourse, image and novelty in the postwar United States also catalysed dollmaking innovation. Gaining a competitive edge in the marketplace led certain manufacturers such as Effanbee, Virga and Aranbee to search out French co-marketing partners. Ideal settled for more local partners such as Revlon and Toni and found obvious success. Conversely Madame Alexander confidently generated quality and charisma on her own initiative. Her transformative zeal identified her as an exemplar of the North American Jewish experience at the same time that her dolls generally obliterated any obvious signs of Jewish emigrant status in favour of the unquestioned elite whiteness of such figures as Queen Elizabeth II, Margot Fonteyn, Scarlett O'Hara.

Such forces established a site for a rapprochement between high design and dolls that has greatly influenced doll production and releases in the last two decades. Although by no means formally validated through the intense text and philosophical frameworks and networks of international academic postmodernism, dolls are inherently postmodern, rather than modern. Like certain periods of art history such as the *maniera*, dolls suggest that postmodernist values have existed in albeit simple forms and parallels during earlier eras and beyond the academy. Postmodernist cultural forms such as hybridity, the creole, the transitional, the crossover have facilitated a cultural climate in which presentations of elite design in doll form make perfect sense. The imbrication of art and commodity is now openly discussed entailing a greater honesty about the artwork's function as tradeable commodity and consumable and the loss of currency of myths regarding the purity and impartiality of the 'fine arts' against the taint of 'trade' and the marketplace. Fashion is an essential part of this process. Like popular music and (increasingly) interior design and garden architecture, fashion is an avant-garde discipline that is embraced without qualm by a general audience. Conversely fashion lends art-and-design credibility and cultural/intellectual content to dolls as witnessed by the recent extraordinary crossover phenomenon of Gina Garan's promotion of the once-obscure Blythe doll, which has unfolded in a transnational community of design and fashion aficionados rather than doll collectors.

Doll-sized couture has made an intermittent appearance since the mid-1980s amongst the plethora of licensed products endorsed by international designers. No longer just made for prestigious one-off events, dolls wearing designs officially credited to major fashion designers are regularly offered to collectors. Such product has a further history going back intermittently over three decades to the 1950s. In 1951, inspired by the recent success of the Théâtre de la Mode, the North American Effanbee company commissioned Schiaparelli to dress some of their Honey line of dolls (see Figure 7.1). Schiaparelli's models were clearly identified with the designer's signature printed on their wrist tag. This range included a doll dressed in an elaborate, romantic ball gown with ribbon appliqué to the bodice as well as formal New Look daywear with appropriate accessorising such as high-quality millinery.

Honey was not the only Schiaparelli collaboration with dollmakers. After the success of Alexander's Cissy, Schiaparelli again turned to dolls and worked with a small American doll company named Virga to market a series of dolls in 1956. One model was named after Schiaparelli's daughter Go-Go and she had two sisters: the larger Chi-Chi and the ballerina Tu-Tu. Schiaparelli's second set of dolls for the United States market were children in the 'Ginny' format, but wearing adult-styled clothes. However, they bore at least one trace of the once-outrageous designer's hand: wild hair colours of green and pink. At this late stage of her career Schiaparelli was eclipsed by the strong postwar generation of male designers such as Dior (White 1986: 208–13), and her dolls perhaps represented the strategy of a woman seeking licences in any media for her name. To employ an international icon of fashion design (even a fading star) was a bold and unusual step for a small company to take. The leap from the comfortable and functional American toy-market into the more speculative and free-thinking paradigms of couture suggests

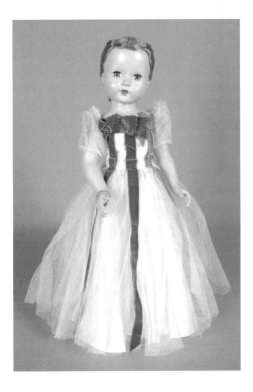

Figure 7.1 Honey by Effanbee wearing evening dress by Elsa Schiaparelli 1951, image by courtesy of McMasters Harris Auctions, USA.

that companies seeking to outflank Madame Alexander had to be enterprising and try out any ideas, even the more unlikely. Conversely one could say that the dolls with pink and green hair are imbued with the spirit of experimentation and surrealism to which Schiaparelli was attuned during the 1930s. Their alliterative, infantile names are also a faint reflection of the Dada or Surrealist fascination with non-verbal, instinctive, almost pre-verbal communication. These dolls are also informed by her track record of receptivity to unusual opportunities for collaboration.

Schiaparelli's dolls are little known. Until recently the obscurity of Schiaparelli's dolls ensured that they were greatly underpriced on both the doll collecting and Haute Couture international auction markets. The Virga and Effanbee dolls represent perhaps the first time that a premier designer has loaned his/her name to a commercially manufactured doll; this is a high point of the Haute Couture and doll interchange in the mid-twentieth century. Yet the general cultural amnesia regarding Schiaparelli's collaboration, even amongst doll fanciers, was so great that *Honey* in the ball dress was reproduced as a historical celebration of Effanbee's dollmaking heritage without any credit to the designer, as if the dress had been the work of anonymous in-house designers employed by the company (Houston-Montgomery 1999: 13).

Schiaparelli's collaboration with North American dollmakers can be related to her greater engagement with the United States marketplace in response to the stronger interest in and support for her work in that country after the war. At that time she opened an American branch of her couture house (White 1986: 213–15). Late in her career her once-compelling name appeared in some strange contexts. She provided designs for the Anchor brand of British embroidery cottons. Advertised as 'designs that every woman can follow', remarkably they included a version of her famous 'tear-design' fabric print from the 1930s, inspired by Dali (Anon 1952a: 21). At first glance the dolls and the embroidery designs as collaboration with distinctly middle-market suppliers represent a slightly desperate act of a former celebrity, now sidelined, but considering the impeccably strategic nature of Schiaparelli's intellect it is interesting that these licensed products empower essentially feminine and domestic worlds with elements of her former avant-garde brilliance. Perhaps Schiaparelli had retreated from the agora, now so firmly given over to the celebration of male couturiers, but rather than retire crestfallen she sought to exalt or embellish the feminine domestic world. Again the idea of Anchor marketing embroidery patterns by a major designer indicates the manner in which Haute Couture haunted popular female experience in the 1950s.

Named fashion designers were co-opted on occasion into the slightly desperate search to lure toy buyers away from Barbie's total dominance of the marketplace from c.1960 to c.2000. Louis Marx's Miss Seventeen was presented as a beauty queen. Her packaging graphics showed her with a trophy and a winner's tiara. For Houston-Montgomery she inspires a perverse, but poetic, eloquence, in her combination of harsh expression and toxic cheapness, 'Truly representative of her atomic times, Miss Seventeen was doomed to literally self destruct' (1999: 37). However, her wardrobe had a more than usually respectable pedigree for toy product, being publicly credited to Jay E. Watkins and Edward Roberts of New York's Fashion Institute of Technology. In the 1960s, even Barbie could not boast named fashion designers with 'trade' credibility. The designer of Barbie's first trousseau, Charlotte Johnson, was fashion literate to a high degree, but Mattel did not present her as a personality to the public. The high fashion idea was taken further through the Miss Seventeen line as each dress was packaged in a portfolio intended to imitate extracts from a glamorous fashion magazine. Ironically Miss Seventeen is rumoured amongst collectors to catalyse the disintegration of her elegant wardrobe, with its distinguished associations, through a chemical reaction with her body.

From a fashion perspective the most prestigious doll that attempted to capture Barbie's market in the 1960s and 1970s was Mary Quant's Daisy, named after

Quant's floral trademark and first issued in 1973 by Scottish-based Flair Toys. Daisy's packaging proclaimed: 'What Mary Quant does for living dolls she also does for Daisy' and placed Quant in a continuum of fashion and feminist history, representing expanding horizons for women and greater freedom. Radical changes in fashion were credited to Quant's introduction of a new concept 'designing specially for the young'. 'Mary's miniskirt hit the world's headlines. Her ideas have affected everything a woman wears from clothes to cosmetics.' The advertising copy climaxed in a poetical jingle.

> Mary Quant keeps Daisy right
> With fashions for morning, noon n' night
> Clothes for Summer in the sun
> Clothes for Winter's snowtime fun
> Clothes for work and clothes for play
> Clothes that make you want to say
> 'Daisy is a smashing friend
> Her tip-top fashions never end!
> Daisy's life's a fashion-whirl,
> I'm such a lucky little girl.'

> (Anon c.1973)

No clearer representation can be found of how dolls provide apprenticeship to knowing about fashion, and the rituals and pleasure of wearing clothes. Daisy also alerts the reader to a range of female experiences and sites of power in the stories about Quant herself. Sadly Daisy's production values do not match the mod graphics, or equal the quality of dolls in designer clothes from the 1990s. Daisy appeared when Quant's fashion comet was burning out, but her reputation and influence were untarnished in Daisy's packaging. Daisy is, like the Schiaparelli dolls of the 1950s, an important indication of the relationship of dolls to iconic fashion designers.

Robert Tonner's replication of the Théâtre de la Mode in a doll-sized collector edition from 2001 onwards was a logical step, as the cross-media adaptation from fashion copy to doll is itself culturally and theoretically logical. The original dresses were created in a fashion context, and if the doll is often an adaptive medium, so too is fashion. Presenting the mannequins of the Théâtre de la Mode as dolls is a provocative gesture that steps into the disavowed debates around avant-garde fear of women and the containment of the feminine, igniting anxieties about how the 'passivity' and mimetic nature of the doll raises questions about agency. Countering the original resolve not to make 'dolls' for the Théâtre works against avant-garde, elite fears of the doll as a medium that is stereotyped as direct and unsophisticated compared to the knowing, abstract format of her cousins, the puppet and the shop mannequin. Tonner's Théâtre de la Mode dolls are probably the most intellectually engaged of current fashion dolls because their narrative is not entirely synthetic. Their meaning is matched by quality technical and design skills. Robert Tonner's flagship Tyler Wentworth doll sits beautifully in this cross-reference. The mature formality of her features and expression, slightly anomalous at c.2000, resonates perfectly with fashion of c.1945. Tyler's janus-like duality, poised between past and present, becomes an asset. Tonner's Théâtre de la Mode series pays homage to the key impetus behind the revival of modern fashion dolls.

With the recent production of designer Barbies, the intellectual and cultural links between Barbie and mainstream fashion, so strong when the doll was launched in 1959, were renewed and finally acknowledged, if only as a marketing stratagem. Beauregard Houston-Montgomery notes that the development of designer Barbies was a surprisingly belated action for Mattel, a company that is generally an alert forecaster of real world fashion trends. Americans became big-name-label crazy in the 1970s but it was not until 1984 that seemingly from nowhere came a line of Oscar de la Renta clothing for Barbie (Houston-Montgomery 1999: 86). In 1985 Mattel endorsed Billyboy's linking of the doll to Haute Couture with the Nouveau Théâtre de la Mode project, which commissioned Barbie designs from inter-nationally respected names. In the same year, the Takara Barbie doll with the anime face was released in Japan under Mattel's auspices in a collection designed by Kansai Yamamoto. Each doll came with a spare outfit, and extra clothes were available. Sadly this *Kansai Barbie* collection, as it was called (Hammon 1996), was not available on the international market. The 1984 de la Renta collection, the Billyboy and Yamamoto projects launched the designer Barbie concept.

When the Emmanuels, internationally famous after designing the Princess of Wales' much-copied wedding dress, provided a set of characteristically lavish evening dresses, some with matching wraps, in 1985 for the British Sindy doll, another avatar of the current fashion doll boom appeared. These evening dresses are concurrent with Mattel's early movement into doll-sized designer labels with the Oscar de la Renta range and their support of Billyboy's Nouveau Théâtre de la Mode or Takara's release of French designer collections for Jenny: nothing delayed or epigonal about Sindy in this case. These outfits were such a success that a second Emmanuel collection was issued in 1986. This second collection included a bubble dress and a sensuous lingerie ensemble in white silk and lace, complete with a tiny suspender belt and a flowing peignoir. This latter outfit documented the growth of a female-driven marketplace for quality, erotic, yet retro-styled lingerie. Sindy's lingerie indicated that women were devoting much of their dress budget to highly expensive underwear, in fabrics of a quality that had frequently disappeared from outerwear.

Whilst Mattel followed the 1984 de la Renta collection with dolls dressed by Billyboy and Bob Mackie, the designer Barbie phenomenon started in earnest after

1994 when Bloomingdales in New York commissioned a Barbie doll, the *Savvy Shopper*, from Nicole Miller. She also designed Barbie print fabric with the doll's trademark and miniature accessories featuring as scattered motifs, which was used for various accessories and garments sold to adult collectors and Barbie fans. Most of the designers chosen by Mattel as partners have a high profile in North America. Others have strong regional appeal in Asia, such as Burberry and Hanae Mori, and address the strong Barbie collectors' market in Japan and the amount of money that Japanese department stores are willing to commit to promoting Barbie. Sometimes prestigious designers provide a special one-off or a limited run for either an exhibition or charity, such as the Lacroix and Westwood Barbies. Since the comprehensive commissioning of designers in Billyboy's 1985 Nouveau Théâtre de la Mode, his intriguing idea has been revived by others.[1] Paris saw two exhibitions of designer Barbies in 1999 to celebrate the doll's fortieth anniversary, at the Bon Marché and Galeries Lafayette department stores. Designers included Missoni, Moschino and Lacroix. Some of the dolls seen in Paris in 1999 may also have featured in a 2001 designer Barbie exhibition at the Musée Nationale de Monaco, Monte Carlo, which also included the childhood Barbies of Princesses Caroline and Stephanie. On other occasions the commission is a full-scale commercial doll release made under licence of the named designer, including Americans Oscar de la Renta, Bill Blass, Nicole Miller, Byron Lars, Ralph Lauren, Donna Karan, Anne Klein, Nolan Miller, Todd Oldham, Calvin Klein, Vera Wang and Bob Mackie.

Of all the designers who have dressed Barbie, Bob Mackie's theatrical designs have proved so popular amongst collectors that Mattel have issued a new Bob Mackie doll annually since 1990. In some years there may be multiple releases of Mackie dolls. Mackie's status as a mainstream fashion designer, as opposed to a presenter of cabaret, theatrical and showgirl splendour, has oscillated down the years, even during the period that this book was being written. Currently he falls within the pale of fashion rather than beyond. However doll collectors are deeply, blindly loyal; their love burns passionate and unwavering. Mackie's dolls are among the most popular designer Barbies, whilst some more genuinely avantgarde and experimental Barbies which show a more challenging engagement with the possibilities and process of fashion design, such as the Bill Blass and Todd Oldham dolls, have been cold-shouldered by collectors. Other North American dollmakers have wished to share Bob Mackie's unfailing appeal to the average collector and his designs appear on dolls from the Franklin Mint and the Knickerbocker company.

African-American Barbies throughout the 1990s apparently sold slower than their white counterparts until the arrival of the Byron Lars dolls (Blitman 2001b: 96). Not only has Lars reversed the racist trend of regarding African-American Barbies with less esteem, but Lars' dolls are some of the most radical currently in production by Mattel. They lack the sentimental and nostalgic narratives behind the Bob Mackie designs so popular with collectors. Whereas Mackie's clothing never quite sheds its origins in review, musical comedy and essentially theatrical functions, Lars' understanding of spectacle is informed by the production values of the runway show and its stratagems for capturing media and popular attention. Undoubtedly these two versions of dressing for the eye – fashion as constructed media spectacle and theatrical costuming – are rapidly drawing together, but if Mackie's and Lars' Barbie clothing may appear to end at much the same point of extravagance, Lars' designs show a more enterprising approach to garment formats and surfaces. Nothing in the Mackie oeuvre equals the embroidered denim look of Lars' *Indigo Obsession* 2000, or the convertible options of Lars' *In the Limelight* 1997. The latter dress presents two different identities. When the coat with its fur trim, outrageously generous gores and bright colours is shed it reveals a simple velvet shift. Unlike the flamboyant outer layer, the under layer is not at all drag queen like. Whilst the Mackie Barbie dresses have only one obvious narrative, Lars' eyecatching garment is the sum of two cooperative entities.

Byron Lars' Barbies subvert any essentialising stereotypes of African-American women. His dolls have bleached cropped hair and wear denim-look fabrics, emphasising and exaggerating quintessential white fears about tough African-American underclasses. In *Cinnabar Sensation* 1998 he even makes the 'white' Barbie the accessory, the supporting actress, who shares the dress of her savvy black sister. Lars' outrageous divas refuse the ladylike stratagems of image control deployed by 1930s jazz singers or the Motown girls of the 1960s. They turn their backs on the strict deportment training and chic dressing that have been used (with much skill and initiative) by African-American women both in the entertainment industry and in the early- to mid-twentieth century civil rights movement to present themselves as mild, couth ladies of style beyond reproach.

A number of international labels including Escada, Hanae Mori, Givenchy and Dior are now worn by Barbie. Dior has issued two Barbie dolls including a some-what staid example by Gianfranco Ferre (see Figure 7.2). She was dated 1995, but her glittering brocade evening suit with a full-length, tight pencil skirt and full jacket, sumptuously banded with rhinestones and beading on the sleeves, would not have looked out of place a decade earlier. Her blonde chignon hairstyle could have stood Madame Alexander's Eva Peron in good stead. The second Dior issue, 1996, released in time for the fiftieth anniversary commemoration of the House in 1997, is perhaps the most successfully realised of all designer Barbies. This meticulous recreation of the 'Bar' suit from the first Dior collection as a Barbie doll, modelled on the iconic Willy Mayer photograph of Bar, makes a perfect return/closure of the close relationship between dolls and Haute Couture. The second Dior doll also impressed through its seriousness. There was no hint of irony or disjunction in the interpretation, nor did any of the components speak of a belittling of the cultural merit of the Dior original. It was the perfect interlocutor

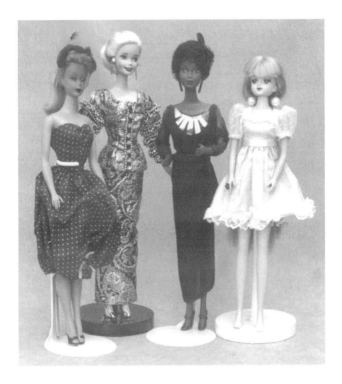

Figure 7.2 Left to right: Number 4 Barbie, 1960, sculptor unknown, wearing *Gay Parisienne*, 1959, by Charlotte Johnson; Christian Dior Barbie, sculpted by Joyce Clark, dress by Gianfranco Ferre 1995; African-American Barbie, sculpted by Martha Armstrong-Hand, dress by Kitty Black-Perkins 1980; Korean Barbie with anime face, sculptor and dress designer unknown, factory original dress and earrings. The same model was also marketed as Takara Barbie and MaBa Barbie and is still in production as Jenny by Takara.

between a dress which has become a symbol of the flowering of postwar couture, and a public that can only approach the original from behind the barriers at a museum and gallery. The ease and confidence of this adaptation also highlights the somewhat concocted and overdetermined nature of many current fashion dolls.

The Givenchy Barbie 1999 is another authoritative replication of classic post-war French couture. According to Joe Blitman, Mattel itself approached LVMH (Louis Vuitton Moët Hennessey) with the idea of developing a doll drawn from a classic Givenchy design. 'A number of specific designs from the '50s were suggested by both Mattel designer Robert Best and the people at Givenchy, and agreement was finally reached on an outfit that had been modelled by then super-model, Anne Sainte-Marie back in 1956' (Blitman 2001b: 90). A long way from the fluoro-pink of Barbie fame the Givenchy doll wears a black velvet and taffeta ensemble in a long tulip line. The replication of period jewellery in faux pearls is particularly well achieved. The Givenchy design is a more neutral creation, less obviously a 'period' piece than the Second Dior doll. If full scale it would 'pass' in any social gathering as acceptable wear today, and it harmonises with established in-house Mattel conventions for long sheath evening dresses. However some collectors apparently found Givenchy Barbie's elegant coordinated black ensemble, with matching faux fur stole, shoes and gloves, challenging. Sadly the doll has only had what Joe Blitman described as 'a middling success' amongst collectors. Despite being 'drop dead 1950s glamour' the doll does not have much 'visual impact' in her packaging (Blitman 2001b: 90) and collectors cannot see beyond that. Givenchy Barbie's '"black widow" look' (2001b: 90) was perhaps too sophisticated for some doll buyers.

The same year as she was renamed from Barbie to Jenny, Takara's Japanese fashion doll was also dressed by a similarly impressive range of major international designers (Hammon 1996). Jenny's debut year, 1986, was a gala year for her; she wore designs by Hanae Mori, Hiromichi Nakano, Pierre Cardin and Yves Saint Laurent. The Saint Laurent Jennies are renowned as particularly stylish and elegant. Some of these designs have been tracked back by David Hammon to Saint Laurent's early collections for Dior. Saint Laurent and Mori designed bridalwear for the Jenny collections in 1988. In 1994 there were further Jenny designer releases from Nice Claup and Fiorruci, with a strong 1960s hippie revival feel, which predicted the direction of later 1990s fashion, and another series of Hiromichi Nakano dolls. The full range was illustrated in booklets available with Jenny dolls. Also illustrated were the finely detailed accessories for Jenny including tiny designer water bottles should she need to go jogging. With her variety of designer garments and high-quality wardrobe, as well as her piquant anime face, Jenny has long been a favourite amongst collectors across the world, even though she is difficult to find on sale outside Asia.[2]

Pink Theory 101: Thinking About Fashion with Barbie

The idea that the Barbie doll has provided a singularly vivid index of the past four decades of fashion history has been established by significant fashion theorists like Jennifer Craik and Valerie Steele. As well as this documentary function, Barbie has also introduced her fans to speculative and analytical thinking about fashion. The more abstract aspects of Barbie's fashion guidance are perhaps less well known than the historicist. In some cases precedents for this thinking *around* fashion can be tracked beyond Barbie to other dolls, again emphasising the intertexuality of the doll/fashion interchange.

Mario Tosa's erudite overview sets a provocative starting point in assessing Barbie's role within the mainstream culture of fashion when he defines Barbie as reactive to fashion changes, if well informed. In his view she has never instituted any changes herself (1998: 58). Whereas Mario Tosa named Barbie as always following fashion, on several occasions it was claimed that Jumeau's dolls set and led fashion and were exported to other countries as fashion models, 'for here one does not follow the fashion, one creates it' (Cusset 1957: 56). Sometimes such statements were made by the company itself in their advertising, such as when it claimed that 'the most expensive dolls including those sent to England, Spain and Germany as fashion dolls are fully dressed at the Jumeau warehouse in Rue Pastourelle' (Coleman et al. 1970: 224). The American report on the 1889 Paris exhibition also claimed that Jumeau had made fashions as much as followed them. 'Perhaps they have even set the fashion sometimes; if so, the best dressmakers of the day need not be ashamed' (1970: 335). Such claims were made as early as 1851, when the jury of the London Great Exhibition acknowledged that Jumeau's dolls 'might indeed afford valuable instruction to adults' on 'the arrangements of colours and materials' (King 1983: 18).

Other authors think differently about Barbie. For Billyboy the reactive quality, identified by Tosa, is acclaimed as confirmation of Barbie's intense knowledge of fashion. Fashion for Billyboy is not so much the modernist pathfinding quest for originality but a network of cross-referencing verifications and quotations that collectively speak with authority. The reactive quality of this inside knowledge guarantees the authenticity and value of both message and messenger. Dispatches from beyond are politely to be ignored. The affirming, authenticating cross-references of Billyboy's universe extend to both Barbie and himself. Whilst Billyboy's ceaseless intrusion of his personal friendships amongst high fashion and society personalities in his writing, disavowed as 'sheer luck and magic' (1987: 10) besmirches his texts with shallow namedropping, he establishes the fact that Mattel frequently 'spilled the beans' upon the exclusive and self-referencing aesthetic and dynamic of high fashion and thereby placed the ideas trafficked around the international glamorous set (as defined by Billyboy) into the ambience of a popular toy. If Billyboy casts himself gatekeeper/guide for those less fortunate than himself, he presents Barbie as a site where crucial ideas around art and high fashion are made accessible to a popular audience. Tosa comes to a similar conclusion about the eloquence of Barbie as fashion spokesperson. He suggests that the reactive quality of Mattel's Barbie fashions makes the doll an unusual and extremely effective forum for communication about fashion, which processes hermetic knowledges for the general public. 'She seconds [fashion's] whims and transforms them into an internationally unifying game . . . [N]o other object transforms intangible concepts – in this case of fashion – into substantive products with comparable success' (Tosa 1998: 58).

Whereas Billyboy and Tosa see Mattel as primarily a documentary voice, Christopher Varaste suggests that Mattel's treatment of fashion is original and forward thinking. He places the transformative and adaptive garments in the 1990s

Barbie ranges at the cutting edge of conceptualising fashion (Varaste 2000: 38–44). However, these transformative formats developed by Mattel presuppose that the garments' wearers are dolls rather than humans. Such concepts as the reversible skirt, which changes from workwear to eveningwear with layers of red tulle inside the grey tailored skirt, as worn by *Working Woman Barbie* 1999, may not work in reality. Some of Mattel's transformations are fantasy and play based, such as the airline pilots and business executives who can add a few glittering accessories and be ready to party. Nor so far has adultwear seen the concept of adding a separate frill to the base of a pencil skirt to move it from day to eveningwear in a split second, as a Mattel package of fashions did in 2002. Whether a frill gathered on an elastic band pulled up over the calves would stay in place during an evening's socialising is another matter, just as whether wearing layers of tulle under a pencil skirt during a working day at the office would be comfortable. Yet Barbie's garments could function (like highly publicised parades of international designerwear) as provocative gestures towards unlocking new ways of thinking conceptually about clothes.

In terms of progressive thought about clothing, Mattel's recent sets of inter-changeable garments and mix and match components (issued both with and without dolls) have an educative and initiative function. These dress sets provide practical demonstrations of mixing and matching, of style, and create the aware-ness that fashion is to be blended and customised as well as obeyed. A few com-ponents can create twenty different 'looks'. The importance of the 'look', as much as the individual garment, is consistent with up-to-date practices. Moreover the multi-purpose nature of mix and match sets such as the 1999 *My Wardrobe Barbie* or the 2001 *Fashion Designer Barbie* is not too far removed from the spirit of Miyake – perhaps ostensibly an unlikely designer to mention in relation to Barbie. However, these mix and match sets often contain very modish and radical gar-ments in comparison to the fairy, ballerina, mermaid and princess lines for young consumers simultaneously offered in Mattel's annual range. These flexible sets of clothes particularly recall Miyake's visionary *A Piece of Cloth* collections, through the variable, non-defined functions of individual pieces and the validation of the owner's right to select and audit the choice of ensemble pieces. Here the dollworld still references current adult practices in fashion, as it had done in the Victorian era or in the catalogues for Bleuette's seasonal collections.

One particularly close relationship between Barbie and the consuming of fashion is the proactive use that Mattel has made of the 'tag' and the label as harbinger of the authentic. Due to the plethora of Barbie imitations, in the early-1960s it was prudent policy for Mattel to insist throughout its written advertising and promotion that little girls demand proof that all items sold to them bore authentic Mattel identification. However, the Mattel label was not simply assur-ance and consumer protection, or a means of guaranteeing that buyers chose Mattel product above cheaper generic and clone product. As with couture and its licensed product the Mattel label had an added indefinable lustre of its own. Mattel's aping of couture practices in focussing upon the logo was one of the elements that emphasised the specialness, the apartness, of Barbie play that distinguished it from ordinary suburban doll play. This stress upon the logo reflects the denseness of the world Mattel created for Barbie: a world which was intended to cater for a child's every need so that her play remained within the confines of Mattel product. Thus Barbie's world included not only friends and siblings, but also real estate and furniture for the doll and consumer goods for her living owners, such as doll carrying trunks, lunch boxes and ballet attaché cases. Yet the logo was not only a practical means of ensuring consumer loyalty to Mattel, it also had a more abstract, less venal function. The logo was aspirational referencing the world of expensive designers, and creating an aura of formalised quality.

Yet again, the nineteenth-century French doll industry had already provided a direct precedent. From the early-1880s, Jumeau's box labelling advised the consumer of where the doll carried his trademarks, and what the various labels meant: either a doll dressed in new or second-hand satins, depending upon the colour of the label. Moreover Jumeau advised the customer to refuse any bébé that did not bear the guarantee of his authentic mark. The advertising copy inside the lid of the standard 1880s Bébé Jumeau box stated *exiger le nom* – demand the name. Most of the cheaper German dolls cast directly from Jumeau heads are unmarked. Mattel made exactly the same exhortation to the customer in the 1960s. Both Jumeau and Mattel seemed to fear that retailers/agents wanted to dupe unsuspecting clients by offering inferior merchandise, thus exploiting the charisma of the named product. In recent years as Mattel has become synonymous with the fashion doll and Barbie is recognised for herself, the advice to check out the authenticity of the label has been put aside from advertising copy.

Another practice and format that Mattel lifted from Haute Couture was the naming of each outfit. This naming is regarded by Billyboy as 'one of the principal charms of Haute Couture' (1987: 26). Until 1972, Barbie's garments and those of her friends and family were named. Kitturah B. Westenhouser, a diligent collector of oral history amongst Mattel employees, records Carol Spencer, one of the most long-standing and versatile designers of Barbie fashions, as witness to this naming process. Designers set out a list of possible names for a particular garment. For every garment these lists were vetted by the legendary Charlotte Johnson, Mattel's chief fashion designer for Barbie in the 1950s and 1960s, who then passed a selection of names into Mattel's copywriting department. The names had to be scrutinised by the copywriters for possible overlap with other commercial licences and to determine whether there were any prior claims to the names needing to be negotiated (Westenhouser 1994: 40). Some names were clearly based upon catch phrases of their times, as well as having identifiable resonances with current song, movie or product titles. The names for early Barbie dresses are themselves a history of the changing culture of fashion. How eloquent is the distance travelled from *Gay Parisienne* and *Roman Holiday* of 1959 to the *Wild Bunch* of 1970–1971 or *Fab City* 1969, not to mention Francie's *Cool-It* 1968.

In recent years the top level of Mattel's production of Barbie clothes, the elaborately packaged Fashion Avenue garments, have again been named. These names indicate that Barbie may well be visiting France or Russia for social or work events, and a number of the titles for 2001 and 2002 include the names of cities across North America and overseas. Certain names also indicate the events or occasions to which Barbie might be wearing the garment. From the evidence of the names of her dresses, Barbie's social calendar includes teenage and casual activities such as *Chilling Out at the Mall*, as well as more formal occasions, the Cannes Film Festival, garden parties or charity galas for example, that place Barbie most definitely at a high social level, perhaps as a young, blonde trophy wife (*Madison Avenue Barbie* 1992 is frequently known as 'Ivana Trump' Barbie amongst collectors) or a well-preserved matron, in circles where there has been relatively little change of values since 1959. Yet again this imitation of couture in naming doll dresses was not Mattel's innovation. Half a century earlier Bleuette's fashions were individually named.

In the last two decades Mattel has explicitly associated the doll with the fashion industry. For example Barbies wearing the four Australian designer fashions were carried by models in the 1999 Mercedes Australian Fashion Week parades as homage to her four-decade staying power. Special collections of designer Barbies for charity or promotional purposes frequently receive coverage in fashion media. British *Vogue*'s two-page coverage of Le Nouveau Théâtre de la Mode in 1985 is a typical example, totally integrated, by the standard of layout and photography, into the rest of the magazine. Barbie's role in documenting high fashion down the years is emphasised through identifying the Haute Couture sources of various ensembles. 'She is no stranger to vagaries of fashion and social change: she has consistently reflected them. Past costumes drew inspiration from the greatest couturiers and her hobbies, toys and jobs, her family and friends have all acclimatised their appearance and attitude to the winds of change' (Kellett 1985: 122, 124). Likewise *Vogue Australia* celebrated Barbie's thirty-fifth birthday in 1994 with a two page article which outlined the growing collector and cultural scene and affirmed that Barbie's earliest garments were drawn from showings of Paris collections and 'were modelled after Christian Dior, Balenciaga, Yves St Laurent creations'. The later focus on a juvenile market meant that current dolls resembled 'baby dolls' and Barbie's 'look moved away from womanhood . . . and her wardrobe mainly consists of hideous frou-frou pink party frocks' (Wertheim 1994: 52). According to the article the 1990s have seen a stronger focus on a serious fashion literate adult audience for Barbie.

Paris was there from the start on the back of the debuting doll's first box. 'You can dress Barbie in the latest Paris fashions' the printed copy proclaims. The sentence is punctuated by a miniature sketch of the Eiffel Tower and a New Look dress: Paris as sign. Barbie's first designer, Charlotte Johnson, attended Parisian showings in the mid- to late-1950s and diligently took notes for Barbie's projected wardrobe as seen in such garments as *Gay Parisienne* or *Easter Parade*, both of 1959 with references to Dior and Balenciaga respectively. Throughout her life, Johnson, a stylish woman, remained devoted to the idea of fashion. Ken Handler, Ruth's son, believed that Johnson, independent, impeccably presented and self-governing, was the quintessential spirit of the early Barbie doll herself (Houston-Montgomery 1999: 33). Charlotte Johnson's fashion literacy facilitated the Barbie doll's extraordinary success, above and beyond the substantial market during the 1950s for adult dolls, such as the glamorous American dolls and Bild Lilli. Johnson's informed enthusiasm for high style impressed itself upon the doll's early image and established a formula that has proven unstoppable over four decades. Johnson was a freelance womenswear designer and lecturer at the Chouinard Art School in California. The School recommended her to Eliot and Ruth Handler as a suitable consultant in developing doll lines, as Mattel had no in-house doll expertise when the Barbie project was launched. Johnson moved from being casual staff to a central contributor to Barbie's astonishing success. Her consolidation of rank mirrored the evolution of the Barbie project, from enthusiastic after work chats with Ruth Handler at Johnson's flat about possible dress designs to Johnson assuming responsibility for the doll's whole look. Johnson and Handler disagreed over the ideal Barbie dress. Handler felt that teenage buyers wanted dresses that reflected their everyday experience, whilst Johnson believed that glamour was the paramount feature. Handler graciously conceded that Johnson, a veritable grand magus in Haute Couture's 1950s mystique, had sensed the direction in which buyers would move (Houston-Montgomery 1999: 32). However, the presence of the quintessential American teenager, the college-related looks, the cheerleaders, the sporting uniforms, the graduation ensemble, the fashions related to teenage dating and recreations, always co-existed with high fashion elements in the early Barbie collections.

Johnson stayed for long periods in Japan, supervising the construction of the clothes, evolving cost-efficient means to replicate the fit and styling of 1950s high fashion in mass production without losing any of the expected aura. She supervised much more than the wardrobe production. Hair styling and make-up, even sculpting, were overseen by her in Japan. Some accounts suggest that Barbie's hands and face were sculpted by Japanese designers using Johnson as a model (Westenhouser 1994: 12–13). One should also note that these accounts seem intended to efface from the design process the direct physical similarities between Barbie and the German Bild Lilli. Possibly this removal of Lilli aims to affirm Barbie's American origins. M.G. Lord both restored Lilli as the key source of Barbie's physical form and affirmed Johnson as responsible for the doll's image. Conversely Lord desired that the eccentric, sexually liberated, weapons engineer Jack Ryan be substantially erased from popular history accounts of Barbie. Ryan only had some intermittent work in designing the joints of the subsequent bendable leg Barbie (Lord 1994: 8, 86). The incorrect casting of a weapons designer as the 'creator' of Barbie[3] represents not only how the doll is targeted as a specific sign of North American capitalism and political hegemony, but also the erasure of women's contribution to developing the doll. With a masculine father, albeit one implicated in weapons research and American expansionism, as well as an embarrassing hypersexuality, Barbie gains a more acceptable pedigree than her actual substantially matriarchal and subversive lineage. Lord even sees Ryan as working against Barbie, suggesting that his predatory sexuality led to the marketing idea that superannuated Barbies, like ageing mistresses, should be traded in for newer, prettier models (1994: 88).

A major change in Barbie's relationship to dress occurred in the early-1970s. Rather than one doll being sold with a wide range of clothes, now the changes would be rung on Barbie's body. Dolls featured novelty bodies that performed certain specific functions. Representative examples include the *Quickcurl* dolls of 1973 whose hair contained fine wire threads to assist in maintaining a set, which finally 'degenerated' into an unmanageable Afro as the wire refused to be straightened, and the *Walk Lively* dolls of 1972, whose heads turned as their legs moved. These walking dolls were an updated version of dolls produced by Jumeau, Bru and other French companies in the 1890s, whose heads turned as the legs moved. *Ballerina Barbie* of 1976 could perform certain dance-like movements. Therefore until the development of the adult collector market in the 1980s, novelty in Barbie was not so much carried by her dresses – usually the quintessential register of fashionable change – but by each Barbie's function. Rather than marketing a series of clothes, Mattel would market a series of different Barbies, each with different capacities and identities.

During the 1980s and 1990s the toy line's insatiable search for novelty bordered upon the surreal. Barbies wore crinolines decorated with sparkly fibre-optic filaments that glittered, thanks to battery power. Tiaras sprouted water jets and 'flying' Barbies dressed in fairy tutus trundled like military 'flying foxes' along a cable. Such toy functions cut across Barbie's credibility as fashion copy. So far not even the eye-catching spectacles of late-twentieth and early-twenty-first century Paris showings have entertained the often grotesque ideas put forward for playline Barbies. Whilst one could claim a surface kinship between Mattel novelties and the new fin de siècle theatrics of presenting fashion, the opportunistic vacuity of the toy company's concepts, when put alongside the spectacular, but intellectually plausible, achievements of British designers such as Galliano and Chalayan in pushing fashion to a conceptual/performative boundary, is sadly apparent. However Mattel's shifting of interest, from changing the garment to changing the format of the doll herself, does prefigure and reference the late-twentieth-century fascination with the constructed, perfected, artificial body, enhanced, modified and prosthesised. Barbie exemplifies recent concepts of the body not as fixed or essentialised, but as the product of progressive modification and subject to discursive, cultural refiguring. Mattel's constant rearrangement of Barbie and the function and possibilities of her body is but a more direct expression of an ongoing process to which many adults submit their bodies by deploying transformative strictures ranging from exercise regimes to cosmetic surgery. The primary impetus of Mattel's stratagem is commerce rather than fashion theory. This changing focus of innovation from the dress to the body/function of the doll encourages both children and older collectors to buy many Barbies instead of one Barbie and many clothes.

In 1977, the directions of Barbie's world were transformed by the advent of Superstar Barbie. No longer demure and homely as she had been in the 1970s or elegant and mature as at c.1960, Superstar Barbie is the quintessential Barbie for many observers. Both Superstar Barbie and *Saturday Night Fever* were born in 1977. The doll epitomised the high camp and glamour of the disco phenomenon and the spirit that infused 1980s fashion. With Barbie the camp, exaggeration and excess of disco were not a passing or embarrassing phase but became a Spengler-esque 'life force' that has proved more durable than even the high fashion of 1950s couture in keeping the doll at the centre of cultural memory. Barbie has never quite left the late-1970s and early-1980s. Superstar Barbie transformed the doll from a merely beautiful and nostalgic collectable to a singular object with a universal cultural presence.

Part of her shimmering, unstable quality is that the official face of the Barbie phenomenon seems to avoid acknowledging the camp, the outsider, the narcissistic elements highlighted by disco. The collector scene conversely accepts and celebrates these elements. Barbie collector culture itself draws upon the relative openness of the disco ethos: any outsider, if he or she could walk the walk and talk the talk, could gain entry. Like disco aficionados, Barbie collectors spend a great amount of both cash and effort to develop their personae and prestige in private. Their private efforts in attaining doll credibility are then ritualistically strutted before an audience, and acclamation ratifies the collector's status and rank, and demonstrates the success of that act/persona developed away from the public eye. In reality there are many covert, internecine rankings and feuds, but it is the promise, the shared myth of this openness, this passport by style not class, that informs Superstar Barbie – as emissary for disco – and the collector world. Disco itself spoke clearly of fashion, insofar as appearance and presentation established an economy of status, marking a newly clarified relationship of dress to popular culture.

For teenage boys [disco] spelled trouble. Suddenly the best dancer in the class had all the dates, and not the football player. Clothing long labelled as 'sissified' was in style, and 'in' boys spent hours at the hairstylist . . . getting the latest razor cut. The style conscious male was getting all the attention. The jock was out. (Mandeville 1996: 102)

With Superstar Barbie a norm was established that remained current for two decades, longer than any previous look. Glenn Mandeville plausibly suggests that the source for the doll's general look was actress Farah Fawcett Major, with her wide smile, her air of vitality and her blow-dried hair (1996: 102, 104). This parallels the manner in which the Empress Eugénie had influenced the Parisienne of the mid-nineteenth century. Barbie's body took on the now-familiar form with the 'karate chop' arms, the twisting waist and the bendable legs in a softer plastic.

As the years passed Farah's healthy sporty looks became overwritten by increasingly strange, exaggerated and unnatural make-up. The eyes were particularly abstracted; pupils were purples, pinks, greens, greys, ambers, taupes, highlights were emphasised and were often painted as stars, comets and lightning flashes. Intense and complex designs in eye make-up, extended eyelashes and eyeshadow exceeded acceptable practice amongst humans, except perhaps for certain rock groups like Kiss. Barbie acquired an insect-like anthropomorphic presence. Whereas an exaggerated, abstracted and distorted eye painting/styling has achieved a much-admired aesthetic presence in the French bébé and Japanese anime, in the Superstar Barbie it was frequently alienating and surreal. Her eye make-up formed a disconcerting, disorientating clown-like Otherness, partnered by the tendency of the smile to become sinister and stiff. Superstar Barbie presented the fetishistic overemphasis of the drag queen, devoid of the drag queen's self-deprecation and political insight. This empty artificiality of Barbie's personal make-up was often at odds with the feminist statements that were being built into her clothing and persona and competed with the valid references to contemporary fashion. Barbie herself – in her body and face image – was self-referential as much as documentary. Superstar Barbie's face, rather than current style directions, was the centre of the Barbie universe. This particularised and self-referential aesthetic marks a point of demarcation between contemporary fashion history and Barbie history.

The 1980s explicitly linked Barbie to certain types of feminist aspiration, whilst not validating extreme politicised forms of feminism: anarchy, separatism or explicit references to lesbianism. There is, however, a de facto female-centric, even queer, weighting in Barbie's world. Both young girls and collectors tend to have many more Barbies than Kens, suggesting a heady over-abundance of the feminine and a social structure amongst the dolls that cannot be explained away as heterosexual. The feminist sentiments validated by Mattel in relation to Barbie emphasise women's potential in affluent Anglo-European societies. This potential is expressed through highlighting the plethora of careers now open to women, as diverse as business woman, politician, fire fighter, policewoman, soldier as well as the more traditional school teacher and paediatrician. The Barbie advertising slogan of the 1980s and 1990s, 'we girls can do anything', emphasises the public face of feminism deployed by Barbie. These careers stand alongside the more traditional fantasy images of princesses, ballerinas, crinoline ladies and mermaids marketed to very young girls. As Helen Taylor indicates this form of capitalist, corporate feminism – rightly or wrongly – is understood at an immediate, vernacular level by many women and is expressed in female-centric popular culture such as genre fiction. Hence her musing over a 'Thatcherite Scarlett' of the 1980s (Taylor 1989: 101).

M.G. Lord believes that the feminist entrepreneurial confidence of Barbie in the 1980s and 1990s reflected similar sentiments held by Jill Barad who was CEO of Mattel for much of this period, and was described as 'Barbie's doting sister'. As a young, clearly attractive woman in senior management of a major multinational company, Barad fascinated both the business and general press and was the subject of much copy (Lord 1994: 8, 117–29). Had the doll herself come to life to run the show? The 1996 Escada Barbie's dress is believed to be a copy of an Escada dress owned and worn by Barad (Blitman 2001a: 95). Bumble Bee Barbie of 2000 wore a bee-shaped brooch; the bee is a symbol deployed as personal motivation and sign of diligence by Barad (Lord 1994: 124). One of the many unusual issues around the Mattel company is the high representation of women in its senior management. This trend was set early by Ruth Handler and has extended to the present day. In a 'long entrepreneurial career initiated in the prefeminist era, she reports that she was often the sole woman present at important business meetings' (Dubin 1999: 21). The question must be raised of whether the singular status conferred upon Mattel by the left and the intellectual as the ultimate symbol of an evil, consumerist capitalism is coloured by the firm's female identity. Could the aberrant identity ascribed to Mattel be informed by hidden but negative reactions to the fact that its fortunes have ridden for decades upon the allure of a toy sold primarily to female and female-identifying customers? Moreover Barbie was substantially devised and developed by women including Ruth Handler, Charlotte Johnson, Carole Spencer, Martha Armstrong-Hand and Joyce Clark and produced by a company with a uniquely long history of female senior executives.

M.G. Lord plausibly asserts that the prosecution of Ruth Handler for tax fraud in the early-1970s was specially targeted at her as a high-profile woman in business in order to mark a disapproval of women in business generally as well as her own personal status and ambition (1994: 91, 94). What her company did was standard North American business practice of the era and went unpunished on innumerable occasions. Handler was ousted from Mattel and diagnosed with breast cancer, a double knock-out blow that could have stopped many women. However she survived both prosecution and mastectomy and went on to amass a second fortune by designing and producing improved breast prostheses having been disgusted by those offered to her after the operation. In developing her range of products, Handler emphasised a comfort and naturalness never before offered to post-operative women. She experimented with shape, pattern drafts, fabrics and fillings – including silicone external to the body – to produce a range of prostheses that were soft, non-conical and had a contour and texture that resembled the breasts they replaced. Unlike other prostheses, hard and symmetrical, straight out of girlie art, Handler's were differently orientated – right and left. Up to that date there was nothing like Handler's product on the market (Lord 1994: 95–9). These holistic, healing breasts were designed by the same woman who signed off the Barbie breast, now frequently denounced as hard, uncaring, exaggerated and serving only a masculinist fantasy. Many of the feminists who loathe Barbie's breasts may well have had cause, down the years, to appreciate Ruth Handler's ground-breaking rethink of breast prosthesis design without realising that the same woman was responsible for these opposed representations of the breast. Handler's innovative thinking and determination in bringing her ideas into production as commodities launched both Barbie and a revolutionary approach to promoting female comfort and self-confidence. Handler survived her mastectomy for nearly three decades, only dying in 2002.

Valerie Steele (qtd Levinthal 1998: 11) suggests that the play function of modern Barbies or post-1970s Barbies – that is pinkbox Barbies though she does not use that term – undercuts the documentary clarity of fashionable style that so obviously commends early Barbies as cultural objects. I would suggest rather that valid reflections of current fashion are found in non-collector Barbies *alongside* the fairy, princess, ballerina, mermaid, 'hair play' lines that are intended for a juvenile audience. Some of the most effective documentations of 1990s fashion in doll form are actually found in the pinkbox Barbies intended for the family toymarket rather than the adult collector. Their wardrobe includes shrugs, boob tubes, miniskirts worn over longer skirts or leggings, wraps and sarongs also frequently worn with trousers or other skirts, camouflage prints, crop tops, asymmetrical t-shirts, bare midriffs, leather/vinyl garments, military detailings – insignia, toggles and draws-trings – all-weather and protective fabrics, fake furs and animal prints from ocelot to dalmation. All these items featured during the 1990s in high and medium-level fashion for adults, but barely made an impact on expensive dolls specifically marketed as 'fashion models' during the decade.

Certain pinkbox Barbies of the late-1990s and early-2000s period emphasise a more feral femininity, and are supplied with removable tattoos or beads for 'Afri-can' braiding, suggesting a greater community acceptance of such embellishment when framing a concept of 'beauty'. Vernacular interest in 'wild' femininity and reclaiming of archetypes of woman as natural and beyond control of civil society and male rationality also informs these play dolls. The edginess of these dolls suggests that Mattel is trying to recapture its lost adolescent market, as does the commissioning of dresses from designers catering for a youth and 'streetwear' market, such as the denim skirt and hooded windcheater commissioned from the Australian Mooks company in 1999. Like all designer Barbies, the Mooks design bore the expected trademarks and styling directions of the originating house. Hipster fashions have led Mattel to produce dolls without the waist rotating joint (originally designed by Jack Ryan) that has been a standard feature since the late-1960s. One model was developed with a soft midriff to create an attractive skin-like appearance where her clothes bared her plastic flesh.

Locker Secrets Barbie of 2000 wears camouflage prints, and there are military detailing and formats such as cargo pants and toggles on some recent street fashions, especially her *Tokyo Beat* fashion of 2001. Likewise military style has appeared in Ken's current line of clothes when he recently acquired some camouflage print garments. Clone Barbies also embrace military styling. A doll of c.2000 entitled *Steffi Doll Street Fun* wears a camouflage skirt and a US-military-style green jacket. She teams this outfit with black platform shoes. With her hard Lilli face framed by long blonde plaits, she evokes the unspeakable vision of a youthful right-wing babe, so consciously elided by such middle European/German rebellious grrl phenomena as the art-music group Chicks on Speed or the film *Run Lola Run*, 1998. The *Street Fun* doll herself seems to be a clone of a clone, as she copies the Barbie clone German Steffi Love. The real Steffi Love also wears parodic military gear in the undated *Body Art* series (c.2002), in which she sports a tattoo and dresses in various camouflage colourways including night camouflage, Barbie pink camouflage hotpants, and a standard camouflage miniskirt and khaki bustier with military oversewing detail. Military references abound in Steffi's early-2000s *Cool* collection of streetwear, simultaneously a subversion of and a homage to military looks, but also an accurate reflection of transnational adolescent style.

Playline Barbie dolls, when not exaggerated by the fantasy requirements of a juvenile audience, reference contemporary fashion far more closely than many of the expensive collector lines, designed in-house by Mattel. Possibly future fashion historians will cherish both ends of the Barbie market – the named designer tie-ins and the pinkbox Barbies – as more accurate documentations of dress in the early-twenty-first century than the nostalgic 'Silkstone' dolls, the Mackie dolls or the *Happy Holidays* dolls in seasonal-themed crinolines – a nightmarish meeting of Dickens and *Dallas*, now so loved by collectors.

Current Fashion Dolls

The most current and irresistible story for fashion dolls spins out around a doll called Blythe. Made for only one year in 1972, she was typical of the cute mascot dolls popular in the late-1960s and early-1970s. These dolls were psychedelic, tripping, in both personae and format. Their modelling distorted and blew out the human form as concurrent graphic design and typography manipulated lettering. Some dolls were home-made in cloth, in bizarre shapes, such as long-legged rag dolls or dolls with outsized, bulging heads and thin wraith-like bodies. Others were commercial, plastic dolls, made in similarly bizarre proportions. Typical dolls include Blythe, the Little Sophisticates with their heavy eyeshadow, the Liddle Kiddles, Holly Hobby, the tuberously faced Matilda and – most strange of all – Ideal's Flatsy, a virtually two-dimensional doll with hair in various psychedelic colours such as lime green. Blythe also recalls the bisque-headed 'googly' dolls made by various companies from the 1900s to the 1920s, marked by enormous eyes and cartoon-like modelling, usually with a cheeky, cheerful persona. Despite her far-out, mind-blown presence Blythe concurrently expressed high style, especially the mod innovations and the extreme fashions of the early-1970s such as flared hipsters, which would be overwritten by Saint Laurent's 'Peasant' looks, Lagerfeld's Chloe and, in massmarket fashion, the 'Gatsby look'.

Blythe could have been forgotten as just another failed doll novelty of the 1970s, however throughout the late-1990s she has been elevated from obscurity to a position in design history second only to Barbie. She was transformed into an international subcultural sensation by photographer Gina Garan through her album and website *This is Blythe* (Garan 2002). Blythe owes this new stellar identity to her partisan, but culturally literate, champion. Many dolls from the nineteenth and twentieth centuries could share Blythe's mediation of complex messages around culture and design or convey the range of moods from pathos to tawdriness, ascribed by Garan to Blythe alone. David Levinthal's photographs of Barbie (Levinthal 1998) and the earlier series of photographs by Herman Landshoff (Fox 1972) suggest that doll collectors could follow Garan's initiative and push the envelope of styling and interpretation far further when viewing and photographing their collections. Carl Fox's album *The Doll* indicates that Blythe's expressiveness is not so much the exception as the rule. Dolls of all types articulate fashion's complex messages about body and appearances, when approached in an intellectually alert manner.

Blythe has also accrued new cultural meanings through the current vogue for certain types of 1970s popular art and graphic design, such as the sad-eyed children prints. The big-eyed and disproportionately headed Blythe expresses a similar aesthetic. When she was launched, children found Blythe less attractive than do artists and adult collectors today and so she soon disappeared off the market. Mark Ryden's widely admired artworks demonstrate how this manner of stylising the human figure has attained a serious cultural status in the last decade. Again Carl Fox had arrived at that position three decades ago, having identified an aesthetic shared by 'the paintings of round-eyed children that were so popular a few years ago' and the French bébé, especially an occasional accidentally more expressionistic and grotesque example from Jumeau (1972: 145). A new wave in fashion illustration that is youth orientated and imitates lowbrow commercial art of the 1960s and the current interest shown in fashions of the late-1960s and 1970s also inform Blythe's popularity.

The revival of Blythe amongst the design-literate has fostered the production of Blythe clones. Dolls such as the Bratz, We Teens and the Lil' Divas have become extraordinarily popular even as this book is being written. The craze for these dolls suggests that dolls per se may become a fashionable novelty amongst the general public in the way that they were in the 1920s. Certainly dolls houses, which do attract – especially in Britain – a more cerebral and sober collector audience than dolls, are becoming popular amongst the style-conscious and fashionable elites as they once were in seventeenth-century Holland. In November 2001 *Australian Style* magazine presented a series of photographs in the article 'Baby Doll', in which dolls were the almost straight, but faintly surreal, accessories to the models, thus presenting the doll as fashion item rather than a collectable or a toy (Kennard 2001: 88–94). With nostalgia for the patterns and textures of postwar middle-class, upper working-class and suburban lifestyles of the 1960s becoming respectable in terms of artworks, design and styling, dolls can evoke a whole universe of style inflections that were once banished by the elite and avant-garde. Back in the 1960s Fox applauded the doll for his or her groundedness in the crudity of basic human emotions and his or her cultural earthiness, suggesting that dolls belonged to new inclusive, democratic and responsive strategies of generating aesthetic validation (1972: 49–55). Could fashion, as the most alert of the arts, and able to respond quickly to new influences, find a useful partner in dolls as the most transparent and emotionally limpid of art genres?

Fox happily accepted the new role of non-conventional visions, the formalised, the abstracted, the grotesque and distorted alongside the obviously white, classical and beautiful in representation of human images, thus validating diverse, lateral, non-Eurocentric practices as well as popular culture. He claimed that non-mimetic representation was made respectable and conservative by the 1960s through the vast profits that cartoon tie-ins in the form of dolls and toys could make for American companies (1972: 37–8). Blythe and other mascot dolls of the 1960s and 1970s demonstrate the integration of a more experimental and outrageous approach to line and design into the capitalist marketplace. However it is only in recent years that the power and influence of this commercialised modernism has been acknowledged and accepted alongside the formalist and purist 'fine art' end of the spectrum. The revival of 1960s mod and pop in fashion, the Blythe revival and the emergence of the Bratz dolls and their clones mark a greater honesty about the boundaries of couth and uncouth in visual styling, the role of commercial artforms in shaping visual experience and the integration of the 'pure' fine arts and avant-garde with the lawlessness of the marketplace.

The Fashion Doll

Fashion dolls demonstrate that non-conventional authorities and influences are now directing dress and taste. The Japanese tradition of anime and manga cartoon graphics with an intended adult audience also has influenced the anti-real, anti-mimetic tendency of current fashion dolls. These new-style fashion dolls also indicate the currently growing influence of Asian styling and reinterpretations of mod graphics and fashion formats in general Anglo-European popular culture. Asia's presence in the general fashion marketplace is not simply as a source of cheap machinists and assemblers, or the old-time brocade and happy coat borrowings; current Asian trends have brought new popular cultural dynamics into play. Chinese massmarket fashion is exported throughout the Asia-Pacific region, including Australia, making outrageous, pop star style fashion, as well as pastiches of avant-garde Japanese or European designers, affordable at the very lowest pricepoint. Eurocentric massmarket fashion has traditionally 'protected' the ordinary customer by 'quarantining' him or her from the excesses of designers. This policy, whilst paternalistic in assuming the limitations of the ordinary customer, is also a prudent economic strategy. This massive export of outrageous budget fashions from Asia has turned these expected practices of careful blandness on their heads.

Not unexpectedly Blythe has found an enthusiastic audience in Asia. As with Barbie and French bébés, Japanese collectors have been particular champions of Blythe. She has starred at least twice at the Parco department store, Tokyo, which had previously presented other extreme interpretations of looks and appearances such as Blythe's human alter ego, Leigh Bowery, in pushing the boundaries of the physically beautiful in an art and fashion context. Parco presented a Blythe Christmas in December 2000 and repeated a seasonal theme in May–June 2001 with 'Get! Parco Summer 2001'. On both occasions the store was 'plastered with Blythe posters inside and out' (Matsumoto and Hagiwara 2001: 86). In 2001 Takara released Blythe in Japan in a new design-literate edition, wearing such iconic fashions of the 1960s as a neo-Saint Laurent Mondrian dress. Fans camped outside Parco department store to obtain these very limited edition dolls and they sold out within a day (2001: 86). Blythe has also shared her beauty secrets with North American women when she starred in a cosmetics marketing campaign for the Nordstrom stores in 2001.

In c.2001–2002 the Blythe clones such as Bratz have done the impossible and made the same inroads into the toymarket as Gene made in the mid-1990s to the Barbie collector market. According to the Melbourne *Age* data collected for the toy industry showed that in June 2002 88 per cent of doll sales in Australia were for Bratz dolls, thus reducing Barbie's share to a remarkably low 12 per cent. Even though Barbie sales had returned to 22 per cent of the new dollmarket by November 2002 (Morgan and Moses 2002: 7) this reduction of the market share reversed Barbie's domination of consumer preference that had stayed good for an extraordinary forty-three years from 1959 to 2002. Mattel has had to implement the greatest physical change ever made in the Barbie line since 1959 by rapidly developing and presenting the My Scene collection of dolls in 2002. The extent of the Bratz's challenge is measured by the radical modification of the Barbie design paradigms. Such an extreme change of shape and proportion is without precedent even in Barbie's complex, multilayered universe. My Scene dolls have the standard Barbie body but alter the expected proportions of the doll with large, remodelled heads, cat-like, almond-shaped anime eyes and full lips. Claire Morgan and Alexa Moses summed up the new Barbie look as 'think Spice Girls and Japanese animation' (Morgan and Moses 2002: 7).

Currently in another shift, Mattel seems to be consciously appealing to young adults with a general interest in style and the avant-garde *beyond* traditional doll collectors – the *Dazed and Confused* and *Wallpaper* readers. Thus the company seeks to tap into a marketplace that has hitherto resisted buying dolls, even antique dolls. Despite prices fetched at auction, names such as Jumeau and Bru do not cut the same ice as Morris and Gallé. New Barbies obviously reference signs of fashionability, defined at a high level of cultural literacy, without the expected romantic elements. Even the packaging of the 2003 *Modern Circle* dolls moves beyond expected formats. Triangular perspex boxes lend a sophisticated, architectural, even artspace, feel to the dolls' presentation. Less 'cute' than the My Scene dolls, they feature edgy styling and hairdressing and new naturalistic and non-schematised face sculptings. Concurrently with the hip hop inspired multiethnic Flavva dolls, Mattel is addressing another economic group that has resisted clean and pretty images of whitebread dolls. The Bratz speak to a very wide range of social classes and Mattel is forced to develop several different dolls to counter their appeal.

Like the *Modern Circle* Barbies of 2003, the My Scene dolls are pitched to an older market than the toymarket, even referencing the young professional women who are fans of *Sex and the City*. The advertising is knowing and urban, representing the dolls as young women with careers and love lives. Nothing more different can be imagined to Blondinet Davranches' 1860s universe of beautiful clothes, piety and family responsibilities in her chateau near Rouen. Yet both Blondinet and the My Scene dolls are sisters, in that both would disdain the repetitive housework and nurturing duties implied by the baby dolls advocated by imperialists, educationalists, alienists, doctors, psychiatrists and psychologists in the early-twentieth century and onwards. Through the authority of style the My Scene dolls and Blondinet both present an image of woman taking her rightful place in the public arena. Even doll collectors' magazines seem to grasp the moment of the flow tide in dolls and suggest that the Bratz dolls and their peers such as the Get Real Girls, the My Scene Barbies and the sudden rush of 'groovy' contemporary rag dolls – again referencing dolls from the 1960s – are ushering in an era of 'doll power' (Fitzgerald 2003: 48–9), suggesting that the doll does not mean weakness and passivity but female visibility and empowerment. This reading recalls Stella Bruzzi's identification of an agency exerted by certain ultra-feminine transgressors in contemporary suspense films (Bruzzi 1997: 126–9, 135–7, 139–40). As said previously the signs of this freewheeling feminine power strangely resemble a classic pinkbox Barbie.

If the Bratz, *Modern Circle* and the My Scene dolls return the doll to the city where she was so firmly placed in the Second Empire, other dolls can recapture elements that some regard as lost in modern life. The second chapter indicated how current fashion dolls could console those who mourn modern life and modern fashion's lack of 'quintessential' femininity. However these regrets are not only being expressed by outsiders or those undereducated in fashion. At his January 2002 retirement Yves Saint Laurent complained to *Paris Match*, 'I have nothing in common with this new world of fashion, which has been reduced to mere window dressing. Elegance and beauty have been banished' (qtd McCann 2002: 17). Many customers and observers share his fears. There was much debate about whether Saint Laurent's retirement marked the end of the couture industry, of 'civilisation as we have known it', or whether Saint Laurent himself had atrophied over the past two decades and his parades functioned as endlessly morbid retrospective spectacles. 'YSL couture was considered the last stronghold in a war' against the swallowing up of fashion houses by large corporations and the dominance of money and marketing in the high fashion arena, 'a war that fashionistas now believe is lost' (qtd. McCann 2002: 17). Could the fashion doll begin to serve as a reminder of the grand tradition, as understood by insiders as well as the general public? Will Tyler Wentworth and Robert Tonner keep alive the spirit of understated conservative elegance? Will the Barbie restylers and re-dressers practice hand-detailing and finely scaled skills that have become irrelevant in the context of economically constrained commercial fashion? Could the fashion doll finally outlast the luxury couture industry that she helped to beget?

Notes

Chapter 1: Introduction

1. Sherrie A. Inness also indicates in 1999 'other than *Made to Play House*, the research on dolls is skimpy . . .' (Inness 1999: 178)
2. As a member of three doll-collecting clubs at different stages of my life, I have had together with other members first-hand experience of a number of surreal and mismatched engagements with the press and electronic media.
3. Whilst art historians generally credit Bellmer's inspiration to ball-jointed, sixteenth-century figures formerly in the Kaiser Friedrich Museum, Berlin, a number of early drawings by Bellmer from the 1930s, when he was devising his first doll, clearly show ball-jointed, bisque-headed dolls from the turn of the century or later. See Taylor (2000: 36–9, 42) for examples. The clear identity of the dolls whilst overlooked in various art texts is immediately apparent from a collector's perspective and suggests how collectors' knowledges can augment basic art historical analysis. These German ball-jointed dolls were direct copies of the French bébés.
4. Other female doll entrepreneurs not discussed in this text include Lucy Peck, Izannah Walker, Martha Chase, Emma Smith, Emma Clear, Dora Petzold, Nora Wellings, Vera Kent, Barbara Schilling.
5. Yet again this is information observed, recorded and shared by collectors. Clear evidence that these 'Japanese' fashions were sold in other countries may emerge.
6. Neither of the French texts, either collector-based Theimer's *La Mode des Années 60 Vue Par la Poupée Barbie* or academic Hanquez-Maincent's *Barbie, Poupée Totem* are yet available in English translation.
7. An exhibition with the same title was also shown in New York.

Chapter 2: Consuming Dolls/Consuming Fashion: Contemplating the Doll/Fashion Interchange

1. Collectors' legends claim that these dolls were made for the amusement of Marie Antoinette and her circle. Considering the generally chaste and sexless

tendencies of antique doll collectors' mythologies (as compared to Barbie doll collectors' mythologies) this is a surprisingly racy story. For illustrations of a pair of these dolls, male and female, in full costume, see the *Doll Reader* (Ratcliff 1986: 96–7). These dolls are certainly dressed in eighteenth-century fabric (albeit in some cases such as the gentleman's breeches in poorly matched scale); some of the sewing skills and decorations would appear to be from that era, although the train of the female doll does not entirely match standard eighteenth-century dressmaking practice in its format. Likewise the ribbon-work embroidery looks more typical of the turn of the twentieth century. John Noble (2000: 45–7) discusses several examples at length and accepts them as authentic. The Colemans suggest that elements and components of the dolls, at least, are of later date (1986: 312). One famous group of wooden dolls, elaborately dressed in eighteenth-century silks, that were for many years believed to date from the eighteenth century, the 'School for Scandal' dolls, are now considered to be early twentieth-century pastiches assembled by a London antique dealer (Coleman et al. 1986: 555–6, 1049).

2. Also known as the 'silkstone' dolls, on account of the tradename of the special plastic formula of the dolls.

3. An example of how current tensions between new and old forms of academic practice are played out around Barbie would be William C. Dowling's article 'Scholarly Publishing in the Age of Oprah' (1997: 115–34). Women, be they the Barbie doll, lesbians such as Rand, or women of colour such as Oprah, are here cast as malign symbols and drivers of changes in scholarly practices which are devaluing traditions and instituting new specious, trivial, subjective, slipshod styles and subjects of research and writing where the former accepted signifiers of excellence, dedication, analysis, reliability, are no longer acclaimed. Detailed textual analyses of minor Roman poets are struck off publishers' backlists whereas studies foregrounding dolls and same-sex relationships are warmly accepted in a world where the sensational values of popular culture rule. Barbie's presence is here not incidental but both symptom and catalyst of the destruction of scholarly 'traditions'.

4. Beata Frydryczak (2003) presents collecting as a more open-ended practice than suggested in the current discussion. Through Walter Benjamin's writing she identifies collecting as a fluid process of experience, selection and appropriation, which makes sense within a context of fragmentation and excess. Furthermore she suggests (2003: 184) that the collector moves through the materiality of things in a similar manner to the *flâneur* moving through the ephemeral sphere of impressions and images. This thesis convincingly places the phenomenon of collecting as central to late-capitalist experience and postmodernist cultural formats. As noted earlier the complex culture of the doll is more postmodernist than modernist. However, if as Frydryczak suggests

(2003: 184) Benjamin sees the collector as an 'allegorist' redeeming the fragmentary and imperfect, antique doll collecting as currently practiced in the United States (as reflected in the literature produced to serve collectors), eschews the fragmentary, the imperfect, the abject or the transitory. Current antique doll collecting constantly identifies the perfect or complete as solely worthy of esteem. The rigour of a peer-validated affirmation of a system or structure or aesthetic and monetary virtu and the fixed one-dimensional conclusions of modernism and the Enlightenment are constantly asserted in antique doll collecting over the mobile transformative vision of personal subjectivity or the syncretic, bricolage action of gathering and sense-creating. Ironically at the same time that the public face of antique doll collecting in effect rejects postmodernism to affirm the positivism of Enlightenment discourse, antique dolls – as noted in Chapter One – are vulnerable to all manner of interventions and falsifications of their histories and physical materiality, usually for the purpose of monetary gain. Whilst the world of the doll is postmodernist and whilst collectors may often invoke antique dolls and/or doll collecting as a feminine, romantic departure from the pressures/aridity of the 'real' world of masculine affairs, the lingua franca of exchange in the collectors' world is unashamedly capitalist, possibly because much of the literature is written by those who deal in dolls: Duveen rather than Berenson wields the pen.

5. One notes that Holbrook is the chairman of a firm specialising in the auctioning of antique dolls and that there would be an advantage to all those involved at various stages of the complex but relatively tightly organised international trade in antique dolls if their aesthetic merits were recognised by a broader and more culturally literate audience. However Holbrook's assertion that dolls should be considered in terms of broader art and cultural paradigms should be acknowledged as an argument that is infrequently heard in collector circles, or even less so in the last decade than it was in the 1960s and 1970s.

Chapter 3: When Paris Was a Doll: Nineteenth-Century French Couture Dolls

1. Whilst one could suggest that Wharton as an American is herself representing a stereotype of French upper-class manners, the narrative weight of *Madame de Treymes* favours the French. They may be archaic, but display a stasis and central authority, whereas the North Americans are constantly being presented as baffled and confused outsiders, wrongly believing that they see through the 'duplicitous' French and can outmanoeuvre them.

2. The relative lack of ballerinas amongst nineteenth-century French dolls is a strange omission in light of the ongoing popularity of ballerina dolls since the 1930s, or it is perhaps indicative of the low status of French ballerinas in the period of the post-romantic ballet. Most surviving nineteenth-century ballerina dolls seem to be of German or British origin; the ballerina is conflated with the British Victorian Christmas tree fairy, usually a small wax doll wearing a tutu.
3. The plate is signed but is indecipherable: 'A. Langchamp' perhaps.

Chapter 4: Pretty, Magnificent, Wonderful: the French Bébé and Female Representation

1. See Theimer and Theriault (1994: 102–10), Melger (1997: 40-41), Whitton (1980: 8, 9-12, 64, 65) for examples of these items and Peers (1997: 63-82) for discussion of these items in more detail.
2. As often, the best documentation of Jumeau's wholesale purchase of German Simon and Halbig doll heads during the 1890s is their frequent appearance on Jumeau bodies in undisturbed and unrestored condition. They are occasionally stamped 'Tête Jumeau' or 'Bébé Jumeau'. King (1977: 396) and Foulke (1993: 145) document this phenomenon from observing actual dolls and provide no documentation to explain this extraordinary contradiction in comparison to Jumeau's frequently stated abhorrence of German dolls.

Chapter 5: Decline of the French Doll Industry and the Fate of the Fashionable Doll During the Twentieth Century

1. With the recent exception of those post-1960s permissive models that have anatomically correct exterior genitalia, again an indication of how these so-called liberated baby dolls are in fact more essentialist in their gender performance.
2. Some researchers dispute whether dolls were made in these countries prior to the First World War. Early- and mid-twentieth-century collectors promiscuously ascribed Victorian-era dolls of German origin to British or United States factories. Writing at mid-century, Alice Early (1955: 150–51) cites British sources documenting the manufacture of ceramic dolls in that country. How-

ever the oral history recollections that she reprints regarding the manufacture of dolls in the 'Potteries' do not date further back than the First World War, although she also cites written accounts that suggest that Ridgway was making porcelain dolls in the nineteenth century.

3. The term was used in the account as reprinted by the Colemans, presumably suggesting that the article was written post-1939, or did the Colemans, who frequently gloss articles they translate, actually edit and change a reference to the 'Great War', the 'European War' or another pre-1939 term? The article reads as if it were written in the 1920s or 1930s but is undated in the extracts reprinted by the Colemans.

Chapter 6: In the Thrall of the Dress – Dolls, Glamour and Female Image in the 1950s

1. Barbie's supposedly inappropriate sexuality usually credited to Lilli also has a North American source in the paper doll of the 1930s and 1940s. Printed in their millions, especially during the Depression, the Second World War and after, many featured beautiful mature-figured women. What is most striking is the unexpected close juxtaposition of the louche – the world of the pin-up and nosecone art – as represented by the dolls themselves in their saucy underwear and the world of Haute Couture and high society life as represented by their wardrobe. In a much-repeated story Ruth Handler claimed that she developed the idea for Barbie when watching her daughter Barbie play with paper dolls representing adult women during the 1940s (Mills 2003).

2. The full details of Lilli's marketing outside Germany are not known. In some countries she was marketed as a child's doll. A Lilli Marleen intended for the United States market with her packaging intact and tradename clearly displayed was in the possession of noted North American collectors Lisa and Mark Scherzer in 1997, as affirmed to the author in that year. Bild Lilli's smaller seven inch version was not replicated by other dollmakers. A set of beautifully finished 1950s garments bearing a Californian label, Joanie Kaye of Glendale California, formerly in Lisa Scherzer's collection has been scattered internationally around doll collectors, including the present author. They fit the small Lilli perfectly, suggesting that she was sufficiently established in North America for a dolls' dressmaker to produce quality clothes for the miniature Lilli. Unlike the other Lillis in Scherzer's possession, the doll who fitted the wardrobe had no recorded German provenance, either of a recent export as a collectable or sent from Germany as a gift or as a souvenir in the 1950s.

3. A related series of myths define Barbie's 'true identity' as gay, transvestite or transgendered male of American origin rather than German (Rogers 1999: 46–7), indicating that the doll's visual femininity is not straightforward but mediated through current debates on gender and sexuality. A further series of myths identify Ken as a would-be Barbie, and he is 'liberated' into his 'true' identity by being squeezed into actual Barbie clothes or re-dressed by Barbie artists and restylers in flamboyant drag queen evening or performance wear. Conversely many Barbies 'switch . . . wardrobes with Ken or GI Joe' (Dubin 1999: 28).

4. The original source appears to be a Jewish newspaper from the San Francisco Bay area.

5. The tale that in London Harry Potter fans were baffled and angry to watch the story of a German transsexual when they paid money to attend what they thought was a musical comedy about Hedwig, Harry's magical owl sidekick, is surely apocryphal.

6. The actual woman upon whom the film was based was a hard-bitten pragmatic working-class figure. She had been working as a prostitute with US soldiers as customers since the age of fourteen, shortly after the end of the war, but she was filmed on both occasions as a more romantic middle-class bohemian rebel.

7. The point made by W.G. Sebald when considering the morally ambiguous bombing campaigns of the Second World War that the 'real pioneering achievements in bomb warfare' could be considered to start with Guernica and the German airforce in Rotterdam and Warsaw (2003: 105) should not be forgotten.

8. Information about Beatrice Alexander (1895–1990) can be located in several sources compiled by collectors both textual and electronic. The site created by the Jewish Women's Archive of the USA (Jewish Women's Archive Project 2001a) is the most accessible account for those who do not have access to a comprehensive library of doll collecting titles. It also provides a detailed bibliography of specialist literature. A text-based survey of Alexander's career is Steensma (2000: 46, 48, 112). For a recent visual overview of Alexander's production see Stover (2003: 20–24). Variant stories of the family history are found at Jewish Women's Archive Project (2003b).

9. Whilst the first lady dolls do include some expected icons, such as Martha Washington, Mary Todd Lincoln, Eleanor Roosevelt and Jackie Kennedy, many of the Presidents' wives are obscure even to patriotic Americans and are beautiful dolls in evening dresses, rather than feminist role models.

10. Collectors' stories suggest that Graves had been dressing dolls for charity only to find that the dolls that she donated to various groups as a goodwill gesture were being sold for others' profits behind her back.

11. The possibility that the Regal Doll Company in Canada also made fashion dolls in the 1950s should be raised, now that an Australian-made Pedigree fashion doll has been identified. Regal's profile, market and quality were comparable to that of Rosebud and Pedigree and extended via export throughout the British Commonwealth. They also could be ranked alongside American firms such as Ideal as high profile and prolific manufacturers of play dolls in the 1950s.

Chapter 7: Not Only a Pretty Face: Towards the New Millennium with the Designer Doll

1. The Galeries Lafayette Barbie exhibition is credited as part of the store's twentieth 'Festival de la Mode' under the direction of David LaChapelle.
2. The Jenny doll moulds were originally used for the Takara Barbie doll, the Korean Barbie doll and the MaBa Barbie doll; all three Barbies were made under licence to Mattel with the MaBa doll being a co-production of Mattel and Bandai.
3. For example the account of Ryan's life published by *People* as quoted by Rand (1995: 31).

Bibliography

Albemarle of London, London West End Theatre Guide (2000) 'Hedwig and the Angry Inch', [online] available from: http://www.albemarle-london.com/hedwig.html [December 2002].

Anon (c.1880) *Purchase Me Young Lady*, Paris: Jumeau np.

—— (c.1889) *Bebe Jumeau à L'Exposition*, Paris: Jumeau np.

—— (1947) Untitled (Salvation Army in the USA Condemns Current Fashion) *Clothing News*, 1 October 1947, p.3.

—— (1952a) Untitled (advertisement for Schiaparelli designs for Anchor Threads) *Draper of Australasia*, 52(11): 21.

—— (1952b) 'German Haute Couture Collections', *Draper of Australasia*, 52(11): 52.

—— (1954) 'Virginia Shown at "Dolls Through the Ages" in Park Lane', *Draper of Australasia*, 54(11): 19.

—— (c.late 1950s) *Revlon Doll by Ideal*, brochure np.

—— (c.1973) 'Fashions by Mary Quant for Daisy, the Best-Dressed Doll in the World' packaging np.

—— (1998) 'The Marque: A Singular Event in Doll History', *Antique Doll Collector*, 2(1): 28–9.

—— (2001) 'Portrait of A Doll Artist: Screen Goddess', *Doll*, 36: 8–11.

—— (2002) 'Théâtre de la Mode Survival of Haute Couture in the 40s', [online] available from: http://www.ufdc.org/doll_news.html [December 2002].

Astor-Kaiser, Inge (1999) 'And Max Created Lilli Doll: the Fifties and Lilli Doll, The Making of a New Female Identity', *Barbie Bazaar*, 11(5): 60–65.

Auction Gallery (1999) *Antique Doll Collector*, 2(2): 16.

Bachmann, Manfred ed. (1985) *Der Universal Spielwaren-Katalog*, Cumberland, (Maryland)/Sonnenburg (Germany): Hobby House Press/Spielzeug Museum Sonnenburg.

Baker, Dottie (1986) 'Where is Hitty?', *Doll Reader,* 24(2): 102–7.

Beier, Ulli. (1980) *Mirka*, Melbourne: Macmillan.

Billyboy (1987) *Barbie Her Life and Times and The New Theatre of Fashion*, Morebank (New South Wales): Transworld.

—— (2003) Philosophy of Bleuette. *Foundation Tanagra* [online] available from: http://www.fondationtanagra.com/index.cfm?article=14&cfid=878369&cftoken=85129797 [April 2003] first seen 2001

Blau, Clair (1996) *Hat Making for Dolls 1855–1916*, Grantsville (Maryland): Hobby House Press.

Blitman, Joe (2001a) 'Uptown Girl! Designer Duds For Barbie Doll Part One', *Barbie Bazaar,* 13(5): 84–95.

—— (2001b) 'Uptown Girl! Designer Duds for Barbie [sic] Part Two', *Barbie Bazaar*, 13(6): 89–100.

von Boehn, Max (1966) *Dolls and Puppets* (Josephine Nicoll trans.), New York: Cooper Square Publications, reprinted from edition of c.1930.

Boime, Albert (1995) *Art and the French Commune: Imagining Paris After War and Revolution*, Princeton University Press.

Brittaine, Joan (2001) 'Under the Auctioneer's Hammer: Dolls Around the World', *Doll*, 41: 56–7.

Bruzzi, Stella (1997) *Undressing Cinema: Clothing and Identity in the Movies*, London: Routledge.

Byrne, Eleanor and McQuillan, Martin (1999) *Deconstructing Disney*, London: Pluto Press.

Carrillo, Joseph A. (1999) 'Something About Cissy', *Doll Reader*, 27(9): 62–4.

Caviale, Karen (1997) 'Playing Dress-Up With Barbie: A look at Glamorous Licensed Products From the Sixties', *Barbie Bazaar*, 9(1): 37–40.

Caws, Mary Ann (1997) 'Surrealism and the Art of Display', in Donna De Salvo (ed.) *Staging Surrealism*, Columbus (Ohio): Wexner Centre for the Arts, pp.25–39.

Charles-Roux, Edmonde (1991a) 'Théâtre de la Mode or the Return of Hope', in Susan Train (ed.) *Théâtre de la Mode*, New York: Rizzoli. pp.21–40.

—— (1991b) 'Biographies', in Susan Train (ed.) *Théâtre de la Mode*, New York: Rizzoli, pp.162–71.

Clayson, Hollis (1991) *Painted Love: Prostitution in French Art of the Impressionist Era*, New Haven (Connecticut): Yale University Press.

Coleman, Dorothy S. and Coleman, Evelyn Jane (1989) 'Artistic Beauty of Dolls', *Doll Reader*, 17(2): 94 –7.

—— (1997) 'Marion Kaulitz: Forgotten Doll Artist', *Doll Reader*, 25(8): 70–72.

Coleman, Dorothy S. and Coleman, Evelyn Jane and Coleman, Elizabeth Anne (1970) *Collectors' Encyclopaedia of Dolls*, London: Robert Hale.

—— (1975) *Collectors' Book of Dolls' Clothes: Costumes in Miniature, 1700–1929*, New York: Crown Publishers.

—— (1986) *Collectors' Encyclopaedia of Dolls*, Vol.2, New York: Crown Publishers.

Coleman, Elizabeth Anne (1989) *The Opulent Era: Fashions of Worth, Doucet and Pingat*, New York: Brooklyn Museum in association with Thames and Hudson.

Craik, Jennifer (1988) 'Barbie at the Barricades: The History of the Barbie Doll and the Secrets of its Success', *Australian Left Review*, 108: 35–7.

Cusset, J. (1957) *Notice Sur la Fabrication des Bebes Jumeau*, Paris: Grand Imprimerie, translated and reprinted by Nina S. Davies. First edition 1885.

d'Avenel, Georges (1915) 'Jouets Français Contre Jouets Allemands', *Revue des Deux Mondes*, 16(127): 340–68.

Davis, Virginia (2001) 'Little Miss Revlon', [online] available from: http://www.dolluniverse.com/virginia.htm [December 2001].

—— (2002) 'Glowing in the Wind', *Doll World*, 26(4): 20–25.

Desmonde, Kay (1972) *Dolls and Dolls Houses*, London: Letts.

Doin, Jeanne (1916) 'La Renaissance de la Poupée Française', *Gazette des Beaux Arts*, 4(12): 433–49.

Dolan, Therese (1994) 'The Empress' New Clothes: Fashion and Politics in Second Empire France', *Women's Art Journal*, 15(1): 22–7.

—— (1997) 'Skirting the Issue: Manet's Portrait of Baudelaire's Mistress, Reclining', *Art Bulletin*, 89(4): 611–29.

Dowling, William C. (1997) 'Scholarly Publishing in the Age of Oprah', *The Journal of Scholarly Publishing*, 28(3): 115–34, [online] available from: http://www.rci.rutgers.edu/~wcd/oprah.htm [April 2003].

Dubin, Stephen C. (1999) 'Who's That Girl?', in Yona Zeldis McDonough (ed.) *The Barbie Chronicles*, New York: Simon and Schuster, pp.19–39.

Duhamel, Denise (1999) 'Holocaust Barbie', in Yona Zeldis McDonough (ed.) *The Barbie Chronicles*, New York: Simon and Schuster, p.163.

Early, Alice K. (1955) *English Dolls, Effigies and Puppets*, London: Batsford.

Eaton, Faith (2001) 'Dolls with Designer Labels', *Doll,* 41: 26–7.

Ebersole, Lucinda and Peabody, Richard (2003) Mondo Barbie Homepage, [online] available from: http://www.atticusbooks.com/books/mondo/mondobarbie.html [May 2003].

Ellis, Rennie (1971) 'Take One Bedsheet, Draw on it, Turn it Inside Out and Sew it Up', *Sunday Australian*, 20 June 1971, p.29.

Evans, Caroline (1999) 'Masks, Mirrors and Mannequins: Elsa Schiaparelli and the De-Centred Subject', *Fashion Theory*, 3(1): 3–32.

Fainges, Marjorie (1993) *Encyclopaedia of Australian Dolls*, Sydney: Kangaroo Press.

Fennick, Janine (1996) *The Collectable Barbie Doll: An Illustrated Guide to Her Dreamy World*, Collingwood (Victoria): Ken Fin.

Field, Rachel (1947) *Hitty: Her First Hundred Years*, New York: Macmillan.

Finnegan, Stephanie (2003) 'Barbie: A Model Citizen', *Dolls*, 22(5): 44–51.

Fitzgerald, Toni (2003) 'Doll Power', *Doll Reader*, 31(3): 48–50.

Formanek-Brunell, Miriam (1993) *Made to Play House: Dolls and the Commercialisation of American Girlhood*, New Haven (Connecticut): Yale University Press.

Foulke, Jan (1993) *Eleventh Blue Book of Dolls and Values*, Grantsville (Maryland): Hobby House Press.

Foundation Tanagra (2001) 'Boutique', [online] available from: http://www.fon dationtanagra.com/frset_boutique/set_boutique.html [October 2001].

Fox, Carl (1972) *The Doll*, photographs by Herman Landshoff, New York: Abrams.

Fraser, Antonia (1964) *Dolls*, London: Weidenfeld and Nicolson.

Frydryczak, Beata (2003) 'Walter Benjamin's Idea of Collecting as a Postmodern Way of Participation in Culture', *Información Filosófica*, 2(2): 180–87.

Furno, Pamela (1996) 'Black Widow', *Barbie Bazaar*, 8(4): 41.

Garan, Gina (2002) 'This is Blythe', [online] available from: http://www.thisisbly the.com/ [March 2002].

Gardiner, Juliet (1999) *From the Bomb to the Beatles*, London: Collins and Brown.

Garfinkel, Stanley (1991) 'Théâtre de la Mode: Birth and Rebirth', in Susan Train (ed.) *Théâtre de la Mode*, New York: Rizzoli, pp.65–8.

Genty, Marika (1994) 'The House of Christian Dior: Couture and Elegance', in Meryl Potter (ed.) *Christian Dior: The Magic of Fashion*, Sydney: Powerhouse Museum, pp.15–25.

Gerling, Peggy (1999) 'The Truth about Lilli: a Politically Correct Report About Germany's Most Famous Doll', *Barbie Bazaar*, 11(1): 57–61.

Golden, Eve (2000) *Anna Held and the Birth of Ziegfeld's Broadway*, Lexington: University of Kentucky Press.

Hammon, David (1996) 'Designer Jennys', [online] available from: http://www. dollsjapan.com/design.htm [August 2002] reprinted from *Barbie Bazaar* Mar/ Apr 1996.

Hillier, Mary (1985) *The History of Wax Dolls*, London: Souvenir Press.

Hilliker, Barbara (2002) 'Doll Fashion Illustrators', *Doll Costuming*, 2(5): 16–21.

Holbrook, Stuart (1990) *The Doll as Art*, Annapolis (Maryland): Gold Horse.

Houston-Montgomery, Beauregard (1999) *Designer Fashion Dolls*, Grantsville (Maryland): Hobby House Press.

Hughes, Claire (2000) 'Daisy Miller: Whose Girl of the Period?', *Australasian Victorian Studies Journal*, 6: 113–21.

Inness, Sherrie A. (1999) 'Barbie Gets a Bum Rap', in Yona Zeldis McDonough (ed.) *The Barbie Chronicles*, New York: Simon and Schuster, pp.177–83.

Izen, Judith (1998) 'Hard-Plastic Jill', *Doll World: The Magazine for Doll Lovers*, 22(4): 14–15.

—— (2001) 'Little Miss Revlon', *Barbie Bazaar*, 13(6): 101–5.

Jackson, June (2001) 'A Historical Hallmark', *Doll*, 36, [online] available from: www.dollmagazine.com/articledollasp?artid=415&pre=2 [November 2001].

Jacobson, Eve (1995) 'How a Jewish Mother Saved Barbie: A Doll's Evolution from German Tramp to American Princess', *Forward* 24 March 1995, [online] available from: http://users.aol.com/barbie717/ruth2.htm [June 1997].

Jaeger, Lauren (2000) 'Limoges Dolls', *Doll World*, 24(1): 76–7.

Jewish Women's Archive Project Woman of Valour: Beatrice Alexander 1895–1990. [online] available from:

(2001a) http://www.jwa.org/exhibits/alexander/over.htm [December 2001].

(2001b) http://www.jwa.org/exhibits/wov/alexander/roots.html [December 2001].

(2001c) http://www.jwa.org/exhibits/alexander/dollhosp.html [December 2001].

(2001d) http://www.jwa.org/exhibits/wov/alexander/milestone.html [December 2001].

Johnston, Estelle L. (1986) 'For the Love of the Ladies', *Doll Reader*, 24(2): 61–7.

Kellett, Caroline (1985) 'Barbie View', *Vogue*, 142: 122–24. (British edition).

Kennard Walter, Kennard, Laura and Intiyar, Ishil (2001) 'Baby Doll', *Australian Style*, 57: 88–95.

King, Constance Eileen (1977) *The Collector's History of Dolls*, London: Robert Hale.

—— (1983) *Jumeau: Prince of Dollmakers*, London: New Cavendish Books.

—— (2001) 'Examining the Barrois Riddle', *Doll Reader*, 29(9): 56–8, 60.

Kociumbas, Jan (1999) 'Petite Caprice: Innocence, Original Sin and the Colonial Child', *Australasian Victorian Studies Journal*, 5: 106–22.

Kruger, Deeanna (2002) 'The Deluxe Dollhouse', [online] available from: dolly-kruger.tripod.com/thedeluxedollhouse/id31. [January 2002].

Kuenzli, Rudolf E. (1995) 'Surrealism and Misogyny', in Mary Ann Caws, Rudolf E Kuenzli and Gwen Raakes (eds) *Surrealism and Women*, Cambridge (Massachusetts): MIT Press.

Lalli, Mary Schweitzer (1986) 'Scoop: Interview with the Real Live Barbie', *Doll Reader,* 24(2): 138–40.

Ledbetter, Karen (2001) 'Vogue's Beloved Ginny March 3 2001', [online] available from: http://www.suite101.com/article.cfm/doll_collecting/62028 [January 2002].

Levinthal, David (1998) *Barbara Millicent Roberts*, photographs by David Levinthal, preface by Valerie Steele and dolls styled by Laura Meissner, New York: Pantheon Books.

Lynn Linton, Eliza (2003) 'The Girl of the Period', *Saturday Review*, 1868: 339–40 [online] available from: http://digital.lib.umn.edu/cgi-bin/Ebind2html/vic_lintgirl [December 2003].

Lord, M.G. (1994) *Forever Barbie: The Unofficial Biography of a Real Doll*, New York: Morrow.

Lucas, Diana (2000) 'How do I Love Thee . . . : Cissy', *Doll World*, 24(1): 58.

Lucas, John S. (1994) 'A Brief History of Katy Keene', in *Katy Keene Hollywood Premiere Paper Dolls*, Grantsville (Maryland): Hobby House Press.

McCann, Edwina (2002) 'The Death of Fashion', *The Australian* 12–13 January, p.17.

McDonough, Yona Zeldis (1999) 'Introduction', in Yona Zeldis McDonough (ed.) *The Barbie Chronicles*, New York: Simon and Schuster, pp.13–15.

McDowell, Colin (1997) *Forties Fashion and the New Look*, London: Bloomsbury.

McGonagle, Dorothy A. (1988) *The Dolls of Jules Nicolas Steiner*, with historical perspective by Barbara Spadaccini Day, Cumberland (Maryland): Hobby House Press.

Mackrell, Alice (1990) *Paul Poiret*, London: Blandford.

McQueen, Humphrey (1998) *Temper Democratic: How Exceptional is Australia?*, Adelaide: Wakefield Press.

McWhorter, Tanya (2003) 'Hidden Treasures: Madame Alexander's Clothing for Kids', *Doll Reader*, 31(3): 42, 64.

Mandeville, Glenn (1996) *Fifth Doll Fashion Anthology*, Grantsville (Maryland): Hobby House Press.

—— (2000) 'The Coty Girl: A Fashion Doll with a French Flair', *Doll Reader*, 29(1): 74–6, 124, 126.

—— (2001a) 'Cissy: The Fashion Doll Craze Begins', *Doll Reader*, 29(9): 52–4.

—— (2001b) 'The History of the American Fashion Doll Part One', About_com [online] available from: http://www.marlbe.com/barbiedolls.cfm?edit_id=26 [November 2001].

—— (2001c) 'The History of the American Fashion Doll Part Two', About_com [online] available from: http://www.marlbe.com/barbiedolls.cfm?edit_id=27 [November 2001].

—— (2001d) 'The Making of a Princess: Ideal's Crown Princess', *Doll Reader*, 29(7): 54–6.

Mansell, Colette (1995) *The History of Sindy, Britain's Top Selling Fashion Doll*, London: New Cavendish Books.

Marks, Mimi (2001) 'Circle of Friends Fashion Dolls Take a Giant Step into the New Millenium with Sandra Bilotto's Butterfly Ring', *Doll Reader* 29(9): 50.

Martin, Richard (1987) *Fashion and Surrealism*, New York: Rizzoli.

Mathews, Rachel (2001) 'Ashton Drake's Triumphant Trio: Gene, Madra and Trent are Stars in the Fashion Firmament', *Doll Reader*, 29(9): 46–7.

Matsumoto, Connie and Hagiwara, Rieko (2001) 'Barbie, Licca and Blythe Star in Department Store Events', *Barbie Bazaar*, 13(6): 84–6.

Meissner, Laura (1997) 'Bild Lilli: The Femme Fatale of the Doll World', *Millers Magazine*, 4(2): 60–64.

Melger, Agnes (1997) *Antique Dolls*, Lisse (Netherlands): Rebo Productions.

Menpes, Dorothy and Menpes, Mortimer (1903) *World's Children*, London: Adam and Charles Black.

Merrick, Jeffrey (1990) 'Sexual Politics and Public Order in Late Eighteenth Century France', *Journal of the History of Sexuality*, 1(1): 68–84.

Miller, G.Wayne (1998) *Toy Wars The Epic Struggle Between G.I. Joe, Barbie and the Companies who Made Them*, New York: Times Books/Random House.

Mills, Donna Schwartz (2003) 'What I Learned From Barbie's Mom', [online] available from: http://www.work-at-home-index.net/featurearticle1035.html [May 2003].

Mint Museum of Art (2001) 'Little Brides: the Golden Age of Fashion Dolls 1950–1970', Mint Museum of Art, Charlotte North Carolina, [online] available from: http://www.tfaoi.com/aa/1aa532.htm [December 2001].

Mitchell, Louise (1994a) 'Christian Dior and Postwar Australia', in Meryl Potter (ed.) *Christian Dior: The Magic of Fashion*, Sydney: Powerhouse Museum, pp.38–53.

—— (1994b) 'Christian Dior: The Magic of Fashion', in in Meryl Potter (ed.) *Christian Dior: The Magic of Fashion*, Sydney: Powerhouse Museum, pp. 8–11.

Mizejewski, Linda (1992) *Divine Decadence: Fascism, Female Spectacle and the Making of Sally Bowles*, Princeton University Press.

Moore, Doris Langley (1949) *The Woman in Fashion*, London: Batsford.

Morgan, Claire and Moses, Alexa (2002) 'Bratz Take on Barbie in Push for Girls' Hearts', *The Age* 16 December, p.7.

Musser, Cynthia Erfurt and McClelland, Joyce D. (1985) *Precious Paper Dolls*, Cumberland (Maryland): Hobby House Press.

Nelson, Robert (2001) 'Do What You Like in the Name of Art, Just Keep Your Hands off Barbie', *The Age* 3 March, p.18.

Noble, John (1971) *Beautiful Dolls*, New York: Hawthorn Books.

—— (1999) *Selected Writings of John Darcy Noble: Favorite Articles From Dolls Magazine*, Cumberland (Maryland): Portfolio Press.

—— (2000) *Rare and Lovely: Dolls of Two Centuries*, Grantsville (Maryland): Hobby House Press.

Ockman, Carol (1999) 'Barbie Meets Bouguereau', in Yona Zeldis McDonough (ed.) *The Barbie Chronicles*, New York: Simon and Schuster, pp.75–88.

Odin, Samy (2002) 'Bleuette a Witness to French Children's Life', *Doll Costuming*, 2(5): 32–51, 82.

Ortiz, Alicia Dujovne (1995) *Eva Peron*, New York: St Martin's Press.

Page, Nikki (1988) 'Living Doll', *Clothes*, 1(1): 114.

Paltrow, Gwynneth (2002) Untitled quotation, *MX* (Melbourne), 23 January, p.23.

Paris Tourist Office (2003) 'Paris in Pictures CONVIVIAL PARIS The Parisian Arcades', [online] available from: http://www.paris-touristoffice.com/va/ parimages/convivial_pass/passag04.html [January 2003].

van Patten, Denise (2000) 'Dolls of the Century 01/05/00 Your Guide Picks THE Dolls that Define the Twentieth Century', [online] available from: http:// collectdolls.about.com/library/weekly/aa123099a.htm [November 2001]; http:/ /collectdolls.about.com/library/weekly/aa123099b.htm [November 2001]; http://collectdolls.about.com/library/weekly/aa123099c.htm [November 2001]

Peers, Juliette (1996) 'A Desire Nearly Double the Mythic Six Inches', *Australian Women's Book Review*, 8(5): 5–7.

—— (1997) '"Purchase Me Young Lady": The Bébé Jumeau as Third Republic Princess', *Exegesis*, 2(1): 63–82.

—— (1998) 'In a Barbie World', *Artlink*, 18(3): 30–32.

—— (2001) 'The Emperor of Signs? Representations of Gender and Governance in Popular Imagery of Kaiser Wilhelm II and Auguste Viktoria', *Australian and New Zealand Journal of Art*, 2(1): 42–70.

Polhemus, Ted (1996) *Style Surfing: What to Wear in the Third Millennium*, London: Thames and Hudson.

de Pougy, Liane (Annemarie de Chassaigne) (1977) *Mes Cahiers Bleus*, preface de R.P. Rzewaski, Paris: Libraire Plon.

Rand, Erica (1995) *Barbie's Queer Accessories*, Durham (North Carolina): Duke University Press.

Ratcliff, Mary Lou (1986) 'Queen of Doll Royalty and Her Blue Ribbon Winners Part Two', *Doll Reader*, 14(2): 96–7.

Rees, Sian (2003) *In the Shadow of Elisa Lynch*, London: Hodder Headline Books.

Reinelt, Sabine (1993) *Magic of Character Dolls: Images of Children*, Grantsville (Maryland): Hobby House Press.

Rilke, Rainer Maria (1994) 'Dolls: On the Wax Dolls of Lotte Pritzel', (Idris Parry trans.) in Idris Parry (ed.) *Essays on Dolls*, London: Penguin, pp.26–39.

Rogers, Mary F. (1999) *Barbie Culture*, Thousand Oaks (California): Sage Publications.

Royal Insight (2001) 'The First It Dolls', [online] available from: http://www.royal insight.gov.uk/200104/focus/dolls-text.html [July 2001].

Rundle, Guy (2001) 'Story Selling', *The Age* 17 November, Saturday Extra 1, p.4.

Sanderson, Celia (2001) 'Eve Ever in Fashion: Susan Wakeen's Fashion Doll Sets the Standard for Classic Elegance', *Doll Reader*, 29(9): 40–41.

Sarasohn-Kahn, Jane (2001a) 'My Diet Cokes With Mel', [online] available from: http://www.dollreport.com/articles/2001/my_diet_cokes_with_mel.htm [December 2001].

—— (2001b) 'Théâtre de la Mode and its Elegant Influence on Fashion Dolls', [online] available from: http://www.dollreport.com/articles/2001/theatre_de_la_ mode.htm [December 2002].

Sargent, Lia (1997) 'Madame's Classical Ballerinas', *Doll Reader*, 25(5): 42–6.

Sebald, W.G. (2003) *On the Natural History of Destruction*, London: Penguin.

Seeley, Mildred (1992) *Fabulous French Bébés*, Livonia (Michigan): Scott Publications.

Sherman, Sarah (2001) 'Robert Tonner Shapes a Wondrous Wentworth Universe', *Doll Reader*, 29(9): 38–9.

Spunner, Suzanne (1999) 'The Thrall of the Dress: Blame it On Dior', *Art Monthly Australia*, 118: 14–17.

Stanisland, Kay (1970) *Picture Book 9 Fashion in Miniature*, Manchester: Gallery of English Costume.

Steele, Valerie (1991) *Women of Fashion: Twentieth Century Designers*, New York: Rizzoli.

—— (1997) *Fifty Years of Fashion: New Look to Now*, New York: The Museum at the Fashion Institute of Technology.

—— (1999) *Paris Fashion: A Cultural History*, Oxford: Berg. Steensma, Vicki (2000) 'The Madame of the Doll World', *Doll World*, 24(1): 46, 48, 112.

Stover, Carol (2002) 'Patriotic Dolls Salute Worldwide Freedom', *Doll World,* 26(1): 30–35.

—— (2003) 'Madame's Rare Treasures', *Contemporary Doll Collector*, 13(4): 20–24.

Taylor, Helen (1989) *Scarlett's Women: Gone With the Wind and its Female Fans*, New Brunswick (New Jersey): Rutgers University Press.

Taylor, Lou (2002) *The Study of Dress History*, Manchester University Press.

Taylor, Sue (2000) *Hans Bellmer: the Anatomy of Anxiety*, Cambridge, (Massachusetts): MIT Press.

Theimer, François (1991) *The Bru Book*, Annapolis (Maryland): Gold Horse.

—— (1993a) 'A Short History of Rabery and Delphieu', *Polichinelle*, 27–30: 147–54.

—— (1993b) 'Not Just Any Doll Can be a Bleuette', *Polichinelle*, 27–30: 5–18.

—— (1997) 'Huret: A Side Product of a Lock Company', *Doll Reader*, 25(2): 84–8.

—— (1998) 'France and Marianne: Symbols of Anglo-French Friendship', *Australian Doll Digest*, 77: 3–4, 6.

—— (1999) 'If the Huret Doll Could Talk Part Two: Last of the Successors of the Huret Firms Elisa Prevost a "Modern" Woman', *Antique Doll Collector*, 2(2): 55–9.

—— and Theriault, Florence (1994) *The Jumeau Doll*, Annapolis (Maryland): Gold Horse.

Theriault, Florence (1994) *The Trousseau of Blondinet Davranches*, Annapolis (Maryland): Gold Horse.

—— (1998) 'Etrennes, French Holiday Dolls and Toys 1850–1925', *Antique Doll Collector*, 2(1): 41–7.

—— (1998) 'Etrennes, French Holiday Dolls and Toys 1850–1925', *Antique Doll Collector*, 2(1): 41–7.

Tosa, Mario (1998) *Barbie: Four Decades of Fashion, Fantasy and Fun*, New York: Abrams.

Troy, Nancy J. (2003) *Couture Culture: A Study in Modern Art and Fashion*, Cambridge (Massachusetts): MIT Press.

Varaste, Christopher (2000) 'Future Wear: Barbie Pioneers Transformational Clothing', *Barbie Bazaar*, 12(1): 28–44.

Varney, Wendy (2002) 'Pink Paradoxes on Nevsky Prospect', *Arena*, 62: 41–3.

Vogue Doll Company (2002) 'Ginny – Her History', [online] available from: http://www.voguedolls.com/about.asp [January 2002].

Webb, Peter and Short, Robert (1985) *Hans Bellmer*, London: Quartet.

Wertheim, Margaret (1994) 'Barbie Bizarre' *Vogue Australia*, 38(5), 50, 52.

Westenhouser, Kitturah B. (1994) *The Story of Barbie*, Paducah (Kentucky): Collector Books.

Wharton, Edith (1995) *Madame de Treymes*, London: Penguin, first published in *Scribner's Magazine* 1906.

White, Palmer (1986) *Elsa Schiaparelli Empress of Paris Fashion*, London: Aurum.

Whitton, Margaret (1980) *The Jumeau Doll*, New York: Dover Books.

Wood, Gaby (2002) *Living Dolls: A Magical History of the Quest for Mechanical Life*, London: Faber.

Index

Index

Index

Index

doll
  acquiring 'life' 24, 26, 28–29, 74, 81–82
  as facetious cross-reference to woman 56,
    64–65
  as girl-woman 85, 91, 192–193
  as hysteric 82
  as prostitute 9, 65, 66, 91–92
  as sign of abstracted human relations 92
  as woman 9, 53, 56, 66, 67, 69, 74, 81–82,
    84, 86, 124–125, 167, 173, 183, 187
  holding firm against disorder of Siege of
    Paris 91–92
doll bodies 35, 55–56, 82, 105–106, 184–185
  as modernist discourses of the body 185
  as signs of gendered approach to product
    design 35, 55–56
  as *unheimlich* 106, 184–185
  dictated to by changing fashion paradigms
    188–189, 192–193
  fetishised design 82
  fully gendered male doll bodies 105–106
  fragmentary bodies as signs of misogyny
    35
  genital detail in 105–106
  transvestite 141, 145
doll collectors 5
  agegroups 15
  and internet 12, 14
  conservatism of 5, 30–31, 60, 134, 175, 197
    note 4
  exchange of information 4, 12
  high prices paid by 72, 82
  in Asia 175, 192
  maintaining reputation of Théâtre de la
    Mode 123
  mistrust of mainstream media and outside
    analysis 6
  mythologies 5, 82–83, 90, 122
  refusal of male sexualised gaze 148–149
  removing artistic fancy dress of French dolls
    60
  value judgements by 5, 72, 82–83
doll collecting
  as crossreference to popular culture 15
  as cultural empowerment 6, 11
  clubs 14
  limitations 197 note 4
  'scene' 10, 13–14, 185
doll collecting literature 5, 10, 14, 30–31
  limitations of 30–31, 34, 91, 122

doll dealers 5, 7
  generators of texts around dolls 8
  imbrication in collector literature 8
  prices received for antique dolls 69
doll industry
  as catalyst for innovation 48
  as generator of advertorial literature 8
  as sign of first wave feminism 35–36, 46–47
  English 110, 129, 166, 198–199 note 2
  French 7, 19, 41–67, 69–96, 108–117
  German 2, 93–94, 98–99, 107, 110
  Japanese 110
  North American 20, 110, 136, 158–160
  statistics 162, 193
  supposed gender divide in 35–36, 55–56
  trade war between France and Germany 93,
    143
doll play as apprenticeship to social
  responsibility 50, 61–63, 76–77, 166–167
doll reform movement 98–108, 110, 112
  imperialist origins of 102–103
  led by women 158
  radical elements 133–134
dolls
  adolescent personae in 70
  adult usages of 3, 9, 64, 110, 129–131, 134
  adult versus child personae 119, 120, 134,
    155, 165, 180
  adult versus child usages of 3, 61, 86, 146,
    148–149, 180, 184
  and art 31–34, 123
  and body image 8, 16, 184
  and design history 36, 97–98, 102–103, 112,
    190, 191
  and design literacy 191, 193
  and diversity 24, 31–33
  and female entrepreneurship and business
    opportunity 9, 35–36, 50, 150–158, 163–
    165, 173, 187–188, 195
  and gender 16, 105–106, 114, 153
  and Haute Couture 43, 52–54, 70–71, 86–88,
    111, 113, 117–121, 121–129, 136–137,
    155–159, 170–172, 174–178, 182–183
  and modernity 65, 81, 108, 112, 114, 133–
    134, 149–150
  and perfected bodies 8
  and performance art 11, 74
  and popular participation in fashion 20, 21
    27, 36–40, 90, 120–129, 135–139, 149,
    156, 158–159, 162, 164, 173, 176–177

Index

Index

postwar couture in popular culture 89–90,
135–139, 156, 164
postwar era as opportunity for women 146–147
postwar refusal of women's mission 147
Poulbot, François 108
Pre-Rapahelitism 8
Pretty Woman (film) 39
Prevost, Abbé 18
Prevost, Elisa 9, 108, 113
prices, original for dolls 94, 162
Princesses' Dolls 117–121, 134
Pritzel, Lotte 9, 18, 134
product placement 73
prostitute
  as 'everywoman'
  as symbol in French art 57, 91–92
  as symbol of modern life 57, 65, 92
  as symbol of monetary basis of modern
    transactions 92
  as trendsetter 67
psychiatry 96
  appropriated by doll marketers 105
public health discourses 99
puppets 90, 123–124
  favoured by avant garde 123, 173–174
Putnam, Grace Storey 9, 103–104

Quant, Mary 172–173

Rabery and Delphieu 83–84
racial hierarchies, images of 30–31
racial stereotypes in French art 60
Rand, Erica 4, 10, 14, 105–106, 201 note 3
Raynal (rag dolls) 130
ready-made clothing 27
Rebull, Joan 123
Regal (company) 48, 200 note 11
religious artifacts 16
Renoir, Auguste 60–61, 90
  Children's afternoon in Wagremont 60–61,
    62
  Mother and Children 60–61
Renta, Oscar de la 34, 174, 175
representation of dolls 28–29, 124
representation of the male 105–106
representation of women 8, 9, 28–29, 41–42,
56, 69, 81–82, 123, 124, 146, 150, 150–157
  complex imagery of women in 1950s 150
reproduction antique dolls 35
retailing 49, 51, 71, 148–149

as sign of modernity 49, 92, 124
as sign of social development 49
as sign of the city 57, 92
indication of postwar recovery 149
modern style retailing conglomerates 72
surrealist engagement with 124
retro style and dolls 191
Revlon cosmetic company 137–138, 162
Revson, Charles 138
Rilke, Rainer Maria 8, 9, 124, 134
Roberts, Edward 172
Rochard, Antoine 41–42
Rogers Mary 6, 10, 18
Rohmer, Leontine 9, 50, 55–56
Rosebud (company) 166
Rossetti, Dante Gabriel 84
Rouff, Maggy 119, 127
Roullet and Decamps 106
Royal Doulton 14
Run Lola Run (film) 189
Ryan, Jack 184, 189, 201 note 3
Ryden, Mark 190

Sabrina (film) 39
Saint Laurent, Yves 71, 178, 190, 192, 194
  retirement of 194
Saint-Martin, Jean 123
Sala, George Augustus 64–65, 66
Salcedo, Maggie 21
science and technology 47
Schiaparelli, Elsa 48, 50, 117, 158, 170–172
  Chi-Chi doll 170
  Go-Go doll 170
  Tu-Tu doll 170
schematisation of the female image 84, 123,
124
Schmitt et Fils 83, 89
Schneider, Hortense 42
sculptors as doll designers 108
Second World War 7, 8, 27, 94, 200 note 7
  as symbolic struggle against the feminine
    145
  and dolls 117, 121–129, 139–147
  dolls and war time shortages 27, 126, 164
  female survival of 145, 151
  feminine as 'catalyst' 146
  feminine as traitor 144,
  Gone With the Wind as means of processing
    151
  Lilli as symbol for 140

– 230 –